DIABETES & cardiovascular disease

A.H. BARNETT
Professor of Medicine, University of Birmingham, and Consultant Physician, Birmingham Heartlands and Solihull NHS Trust (Teaching)

G. O'GARA
General Practitioner, Small Heath Medical Practice, Small Heath, Birmingham

Medical Education Partnership Ltd

Contents

Introduction

Type 2 diabetes has become one of the major public health problems of modern times. Numbers have increased exponentially in recent decades and this massive increase is now becoming apparent not only in the developed world, but also in the developing world. Globally, there are now more people suffering the consequences of over-nutrition compared with malnutrition. The major reason for this massive increase in numbers relates in part to our ageing populations, but more particularly to the increasing prevalence of obesity in association with urbanisation, changes in diet and much reduced physical activity[1]. The problem of diabetes though, relates not just to numbers of patients but also to the long-term complications.

Twenty-five years ago the emphasis in diabetic medicine was on glycaemic control. Indeed, there was no real evidence base for treatment from the point of view of prevention/amelioration of the long-term vascular complications. It was recognised that coronary heart disease, stroke and peripheral vascular disease were particularly common in association with diabetes, but the reasons for this were not entirely clear. It was apparent, however, that diabetes *per se* was a major independent risk factor for cardiovascular disease, but how this operated was unknown. It was also known that there was a high rate of attrition from microangiopathic complications, which included diabetic eye and kidney disease and nerve damage. Having said this, controversy raged as to whether the underlying pathology of diabetic neuropathy was predominantly vascular or metabolic and indeed whether retinopathy and nephropathy had predominantly a genetic basis[2].

More recently, there has been a major change in the way that diabetes experts look at and understand type 2 diabetes. Long gone are the days when type 2 diabetes was labelled 'a mild disease'. It is now recognised that around 80% of all patients with diabetes will die, many prematurely, from cardiovascular disease and predominantly ischaemic heart disease, but there is also a greatly increased risk of stroke and peripheral vascular disease[3-5]. In addition, it has become apparent that diabetic nephropathy is not just about the development of renal failure, but is itself also associated with massively increased cardiovascular risk[6]. This knowledge has led to the redefinition of type 2 diabetes as part of a syndrome of cardiovascular risk diagnosed on the basis of raised blood glucose. If we are to make a significant impact on type 2 diabetes then it is the area of cardiovascular disease reduction where efforts must be concentrated.

In the last five years or so there has been a transformation in the knowledge base for type 2 diabetes management. This has included trials that have confirmed the undoubted benefit from the point of view of vascular disease of tightened glycaemic control[7], reduction in blood pressure[8,9] and improvement in the lipid profile[10,11]. This has been recognised by official bodies dealing with diabetic patients, including in the UK, the National Institute for Clinical Excellence (NICE)[12], the Department of Health, through publication of National Service Frameworks for Diabetes[13] and Coronary Heart Disease[14] and various pronouncements and guidelines from other professional bodies including the British Hypertension Society and other documents produced by the 'joint societies' with an interest in hypertension and dyslipidaemia[15].

We live in exciting times from the point of view of diabetes management. A whole range of new drugs for the management of glycaemia, hypertension and dyslipidaemia have appeared on the market in recent years. Indeed, it might now be reasonably argued that we have the evidence base to direct prescribing and the drugs to do the job. Why then are results still poor outside the clinical trial situation and why are many patients still not receiving appropriate therapies? The NSFs talk about equity and high quality care, and although they come with limited extra resources, they should be at least commended for providing such a lead. The great challenge now is to put the evidence base into practice through systems of care that work including encouraging patient compliance. These challenges should not be underestimated.

In this book, we have highlighted the scale of the problem of diabetes and cardiovascular disease, with specific chapters relating type 2 diabetes to each of the major cardiovascular risk factors. The relationship between diabetes and each risk factor is considered, followed by the evidence base for management and management regimens. It is accepted that this is a rather artificial way forward as we need to look at the patient with type 2 diabetes as a whole person, rather than a collection of risk factors. We believe, though, that this is a pragmatic approach particularly since we have attempted to bring together in the final chapter a discussion of multiprofessional care including the challenges facing health professionals in the provision of such care, systems of care and overcoming obstacles including problems of patient compliance.

AH Barnett

Epidemiology of diabetes and cardiovascular disease

The last few decades have seen an exponential rise in the numbers of patients with type 2 diabetes. This is largely related to changes in lifestyle, which include both dietary factors and inactivity. In the UK, around 2.4 million people are thought to have diabetes; of these over 90% have type 2 diabetes and up to a million are at present undiagnosed, but still at a very high cardiovascular risk[3]. Projections are that these numbers will reach three million by 2010 (Fig 1.1).

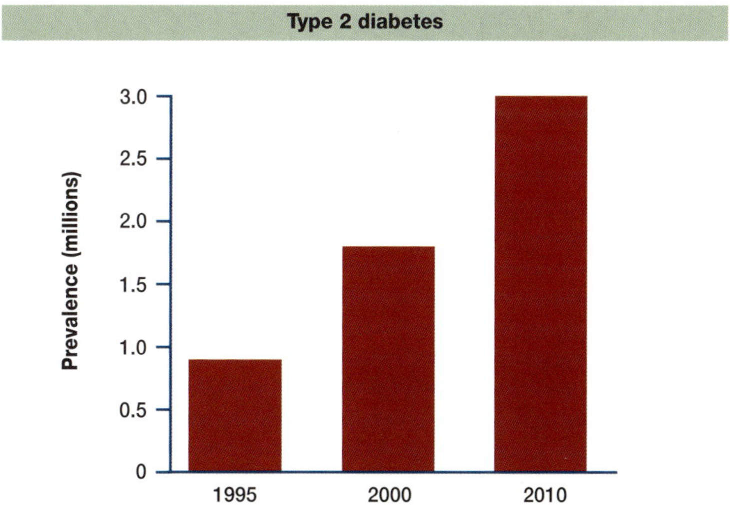

Fig 1.1 Projections for numbers of diabetic patients in the UK by 2010 (adapted with permission from *Diabetic Med* 1997; 14 (Suppl 5); 57-85).

Risk factors for cardiovascular disease

Diabetes *per se* is a major and independent risk factor for cardiovascular disease, increasing that risk by approximately 1.5 fold even after correction for other risk factors[16]. Cardiovascular disease includes a two to four times increased risk of ischaemic heart disease (Fig 1.2) resulting in angina and myocardial infarction, stroke (increased two to six fold) (Fig 1.3) and peripheral vascular disease (massively increased risk) (Fig 1.4, Fig 1.5)[17-19].

Fig 1.2 Demonstrates post mortem specimens of a heart of patient with type 2 diabetes who died of massive myocardial infarction.

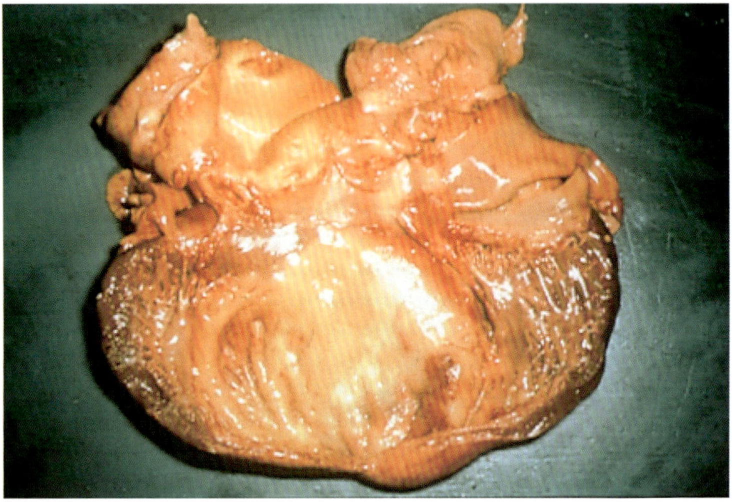

Fig 1.3 Post mortem specimen of the brain of a type 2 diabetic who died from a stroke.

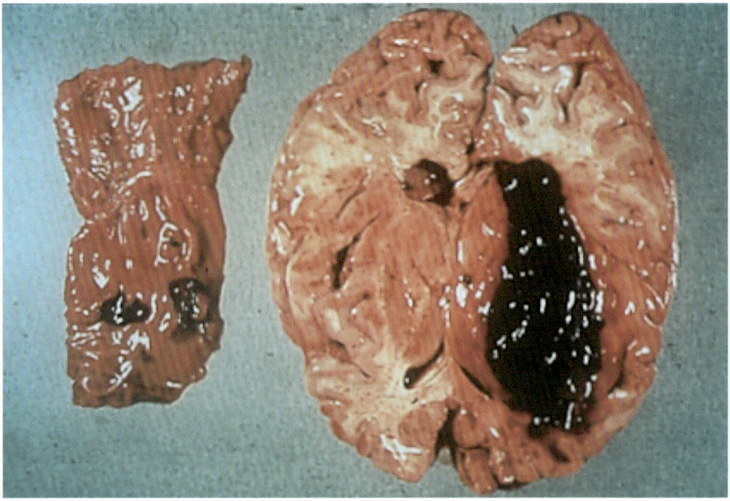

Fig 1.4 Demonstrates gangrene in the big toe of a diabetic patient consequent on peripheral vascular disease.

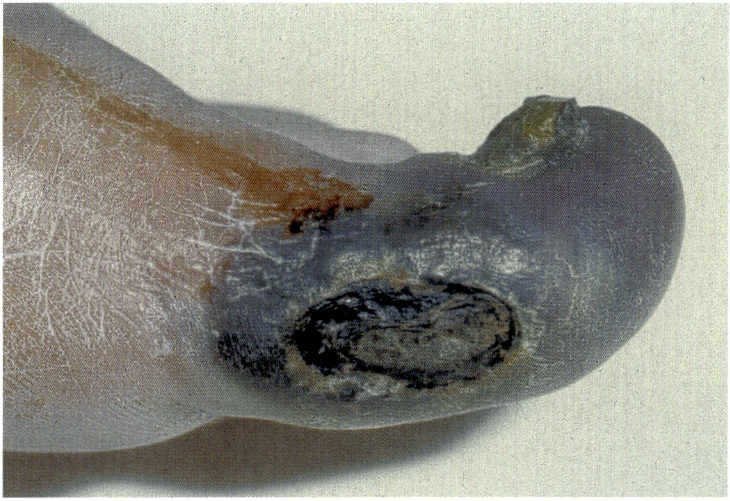

Fig 1.5 Arteriogram showing narrowing of the iliac artery consequent on peripheral vascular disease. (*Compliments of Dr J Henderson*).

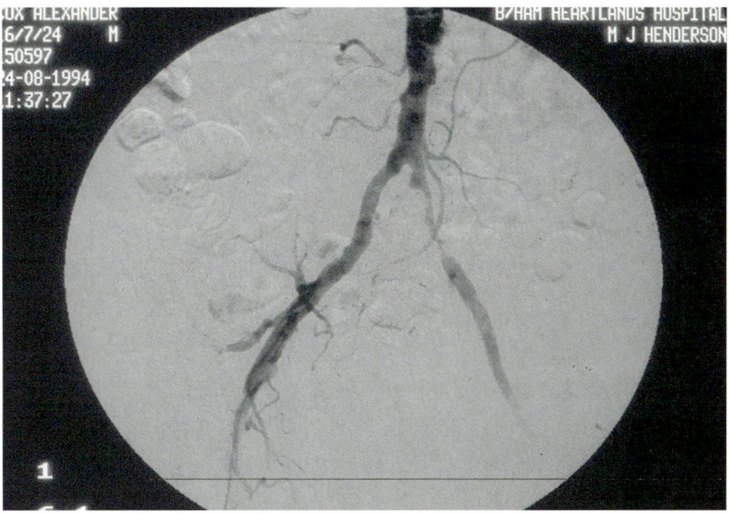

The above relates to accelerated atherosclerosis, which is thought to occur through:

- alterations in endothelial cell and platelet interactions
- abnormalities in lipid and lipoprotein metabolism[19,20]
- raised blood glucose, which is associated with glycation of long-lived tissue proteins in the vasculature and adversely affects vascular endothelium
- further acceleration of the process by the common co-occurrence of other major risk factors, including hypertension and dyslipidaemia.

Raised blood glucose and abnormalities of the lipid profile have an adverse effect on vascular endothelium. Hypertension increases the risk of endothelial cell injury with macrophage and platelet aggregation, the release of growth factors to stimulate proliferation of smooth muscle cells and deposition of lipid laden foam cells[20] (Fig 1.6).

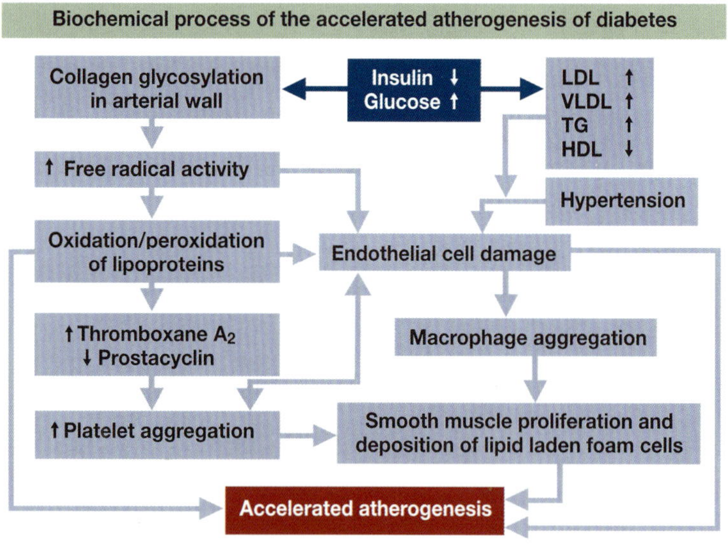

Fig 1.6 Demonstrates the mechanism of development of atherosclerosis in the type 2 diabetic patient (adapted from Dodson and Barnett, 1998[20] with permission from Science Press, London).

The consequences of the above include the following:

- A patient with type 2 diabetes who has never had a vascular event is at the same risk as having such an event as a non-diabetic patient with a previous myocardial infarction[21] (Fig 1.7). This demonstrates that the concept of primary prevention in type 2 diabetes is redundant.

- Women in particular are adversely affected with loss of normal female protection against atherosclerosis[22].
- Both men and women have significantly higher mortality if they sustain a myocardial infarction, compared with the non-diabetic population[23]. This may be because the coronary vessels tend to be more severely affected in the diabetic population, with occurrence at a younger age and increased likelihood of congestive heart failure.
- The prognosis after myocardial infarction in diabetic patients is significantly worse than in the non-diabetic population. This is because of increased rates of heart failure and mortality both in the early phases and for several years after myocardial infarction[23].
- Although stroke is less common than myocardial infarction, it is still significantly increased in the diabetic compared with the non-diabetic patient (two to six fold) and the sequelae may be particularly severe with many years of disability[16,18].
- Peripheral vascular disease is also problematic with accelerated arteriosclerosis in the peripheral vasculature leading to intermittent claudication, rest pain, digital gangrene, infection and the necessity for lower limb amputation in a significant number of cases[16-18].
- Although diabetic renal disease (Fig 1.8a and Fig 1.8b) is generally labelled as a microangiopathic complication, and indeed is the commonest single reason for renal failure and the need for dialysis in the UK and in many other countries, it is also associated with a massively increased risk of cardiovascular disease[6]. The reasons for this are not clear, but relate at least in part to poor diabetic control and the co-occurrence of a range of other cardiovascular risk factors, particularly dyslipidaemia and hypertension in the nephropathic patient. There is also evidence that protein leakage from the kidneys is indicative of a more generalised pathology involving 'leaky' blood vessels; this may relate to problems in the coronary, cerebral and peripheral vasculature[6]. Even subjects with microalbuminuria (increased albumin excretion rate above the normal range but below the level of stick test detection) are at a significantly increased risk of cardiovascular complications, as well as the later development of overt nephropathy[6] (Fig 1.9).

Costs of diabetes

The costs of diabetes are tremendous and increasing[3-5]. It is estimated that diabetes consumes around 10% of the total healthcare

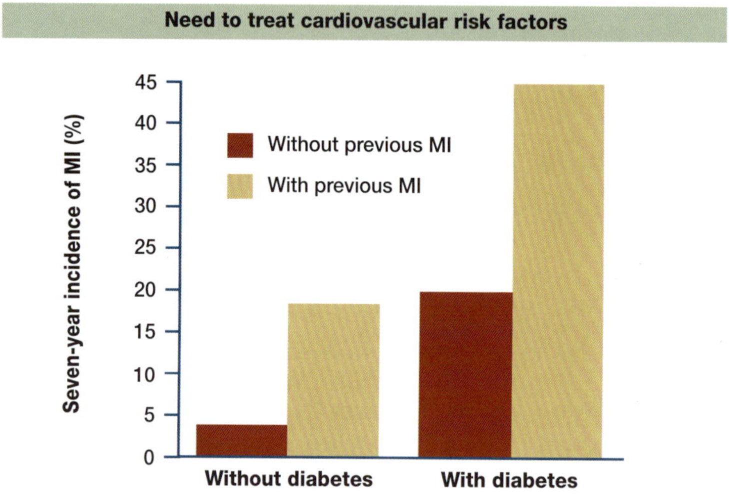

Fig 1.7 Demonstrates that the risk of a cardiovascular event in a diabetic patient who has never had a previous event is as high as that of a non-diabetic who has had a previous myocardial infarction (adapted from Haffner SM et al. *New Engl J Med* 1998[21]).

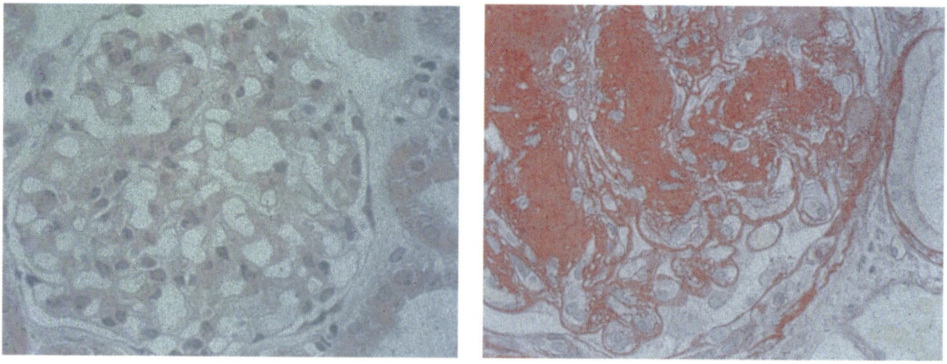

Fig 1.8a Haematoxylin and eosin stain of a normal renal glomerulus.
Fig 1.8b A glomerulus from a long-standing diabetic patient with proteinuria (diabetic glomerulosclerosis). Note replacement of the normal histological architecture and basement membrane thickening.

Fig 1.9 Demonstrates the high rate of attrition usually from cardiovascular disease in type 2 diabetic subjects with microalbuminuria (adapted with permission from Schmitz A and Vaeth M. *Diabetic Med* 1988;5:126-34).

Microalbuminuria as a risk factor for death in type 2 diabetes

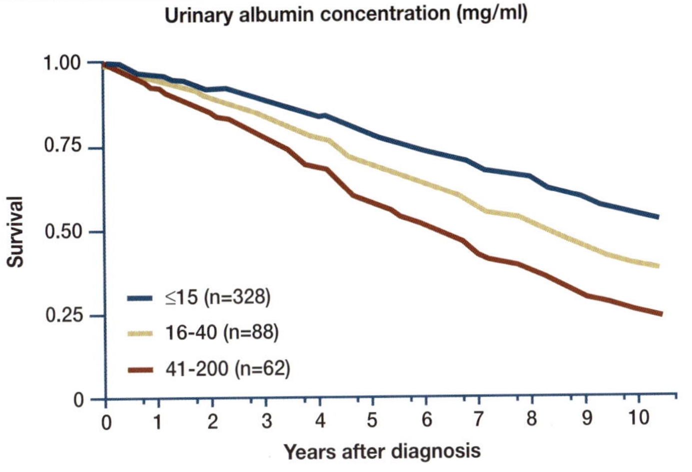

Fig 1.10 Demonstrates the massive increase in spend from the US healthcare budget of type 2 diabetes and its complications (adapted from *Textbook of Diabetes*. Pickup J, Williams G (eds). Public health problems of diabetes mellitus and its costs to the community. Blackwell Science Ltd, Oxford, 1997;1:4.3).

Increase in US healthcare spend for type 2 diabetes

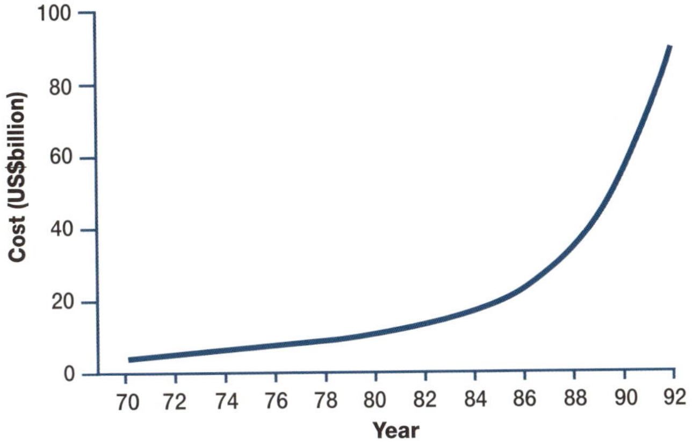

budget of the UK with projections that this could reach 25% within the next 20 years at present rates of increase. The US already spends around 15% of its total healthcare budget on diabetes, the total budget now being around 100 billion dollars per year[24,25] (Fig 1.10). This is more than the **total** healthcare budget of the UK! Eighty per cent of these costs relate to the long-term complications, particularly cardiovascular disease. The costs of cardiovascular complications include not just the direct financial costs but also the cost to the individual, families and society as a whole.

Assessment of risk factors

In order to pick up complications early, all diabetic patients should be fully assessed both for evidence of cardiovascular disease and the presence of treatable cardiovascular risk factors (Table 1.1).

Table 1.1: Assessing the diabetic patient for cardiovascular disease

History	Chest pain, smoking, alcohol intake, family history, other risk factors
Examination	End organ damage (eg LVH, absent peripheral pulses, femoral/neck bruits, retinal damage)
Screen for risk factors	BP (every visit) Total and HDL cholesterol (annually) HbA_{1c} (3-4 times per year) Serum creatinine (annually) Proteinuria (every visit) Early morning urine albumin/creatinine ratio (or AER-timed overnight) (annually) ECG CHD risk assessment (annually)
If indicated echocardiogram, exercise ECG, chest X-ray, renal ultrasound	

LVH = left ventricular hypertrophy AER = albumin excretion rate

KEY LEARNING POINTS

- The number of patients with diabetes is increasing exponentially worldwide and principally relates to sedentary lifestyle and obesity
- Type 2 diabetes is an important primary risk factor for cardiovascular disease
- People with type 2 diabetes are two to four times more likely to develop cardiovascular disease than people without diabetes
- The costs for diabetes are increasing and relate in part to the considerable costs of long-term complications, particularly cardiovascular disease
- Patients with diabetes should be assessed for the presence of treatable cardiovascular risk factors (eg hypertension, dyslipidaemia, cigarette smoking)

2 Diabetes, obesity and cardiovascular disease

Development of type 2 diabetes: the metabolic syndrome

The common co-occurrence of a range of cardiovascular risk factors in the same patient has been recognised for many years. In 1988 Gerry Reaven in the US first proposed that this might relate to a single underlying abnormality, that of insulin resistance[26]. This is defined as resistance of the body to the biological actions of insulin and is a central feature of what he described as the 'syndrome X' hypothesis, now more commonly called the 'metabolic syndrome' (Fig 2.1). He suggested that insulin resistance would lead to the development of hyperinsulinaemia. Hyperinsulinaemia is associated with a dyslipidaemic lipid profile with increases in low- and very low-density lipoproteins (LDL and VLDL) and reduced levels of the anti-atherogenic high-density lipoprotein (HDL) – essentially a profile of raised triglycerides and low HDL.

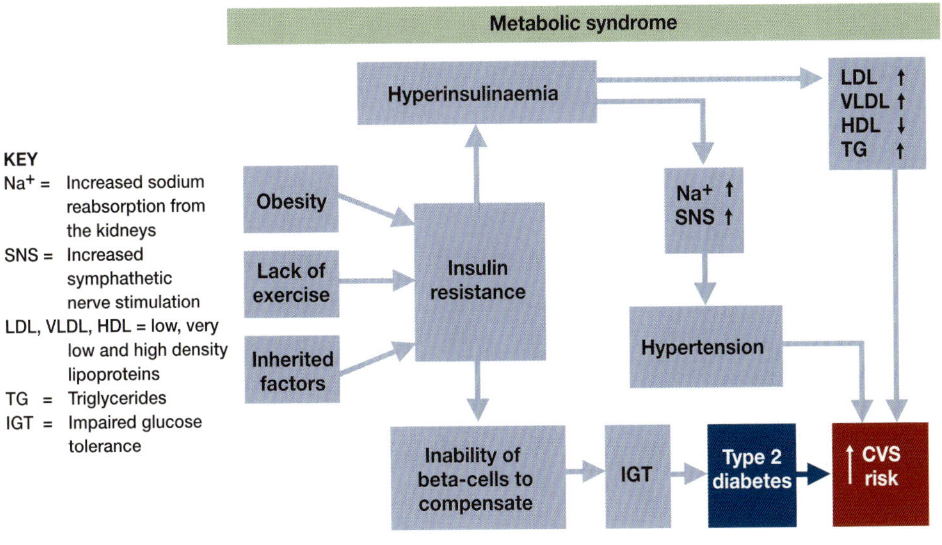

Fig 2.1 Demonstrates the metabolic syndrome hypothesis relating the co-occurrence of cardiovascular risk factors in the same patient postulated to arise from a primary underlying abnormality of insulin resistance, the major arbiters of which are sedentary lifestyle and obesity (particularly central obesity).

Hyperinsulinaemia is also associated with increased sympathetic nervous system stimulation and sodium retention. Reaven suggested that this might be related to the increased prevalence of hypertension seen in this condition. He further postulated that, in a proportion of people, there would eventually be an inability of the beta-cells of the pancreas to overcome insulin resistance, with the development of impaired glucose tolerance, followed by type 2 diabetes.

In more recent years, a number of other factors have been added to the syndrome such as endothelial cell dysfunction/microalbuminuria, clotting abnormalities and markers of inflammation.

It is perhaps not too surprising that the major arbiters of insulin resistance are obesity and reduced physical activity, although genetic factors are also likely to be involved. In recent decades, the population of the UK and many other countries has become more sedentary with massive reductions in physical activity. This has coincided with an increased intake of high fat and high sugar foods, although total caloric intake has not increased. The problem is of particular concern in children where childhood obesity is now reaching epidemic proportions[27], with around 20% of today's teenagers clinically obese (Fig 2.2).

The 'metabolic syndrome', which the authors believe is better termed 'the syndrome of chronic cardiovascular risk', now affects

Childhood obesity in the UK

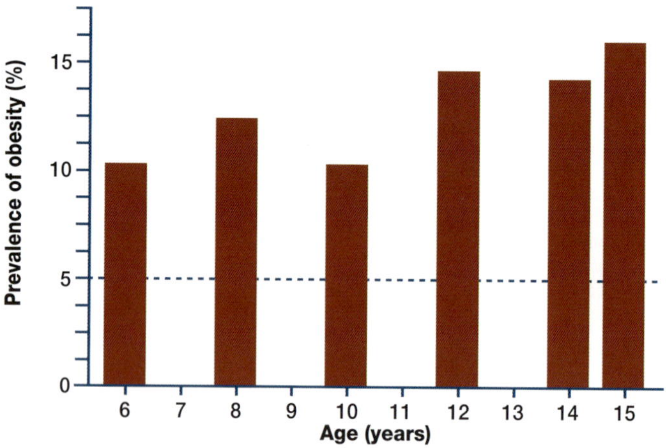

Fig 2.2 Demonstrates the very high rate of obesity in children in the UK – note that this data is now somewhat out of date with figures estimated to be around 20% of teenage children (adapted from Reilly JJ et al. *Lancet* 1999;354:1874-75 with permission from Elsevier).

Box 2.1 NCEP ATPIII criteria for metabolic syndrome (adapted from NCEP Expert Panel, National Institute of Health, 2002[29]).

Metabolic syndrome defined as ≥3 of the following NCEP ATPIII criteria:
Waist circumference >102cm (men) or 88cm (women)
Triglycerides ≥1.7mmol/l
HDL cholesterol <1mmol/l (men) or <1.3mmol/l (women)
Blood pressure ≥130/85mmHg
Fasting plasma glucose ≥6.1mmol/l

around 25% of the US and UK populations[28]. (Fig 2.3, Fig 2.4). It has been defined by a number of bodies, including those in the US (Box 2.1) and the World Health Organization (WHO)[29,30].

Obesity and the metabolic syndrome

Although obesity is intimately associated with the development of the metabolic syndrome, an even more important risk factor is central adiposity[31,32]. This has been variously labelled as 'big belly' obesity or 'apple-shaped distribution of fat'. Waist circumference is a good surrogate for the amount of intra-abdominal fat. If a man has a waist circumference of more than 100cm (40 inches) or a woman more than 88cm (35 inches) then they are commonly insulin resistant with a significantly increased risk of diabetes and cardiovascular disease. Intra-abdominal fat is metabolically active and is strongly associated with the development of insulin resistance. The reason for this association is not entirely clear and is the subject of ongoing research.

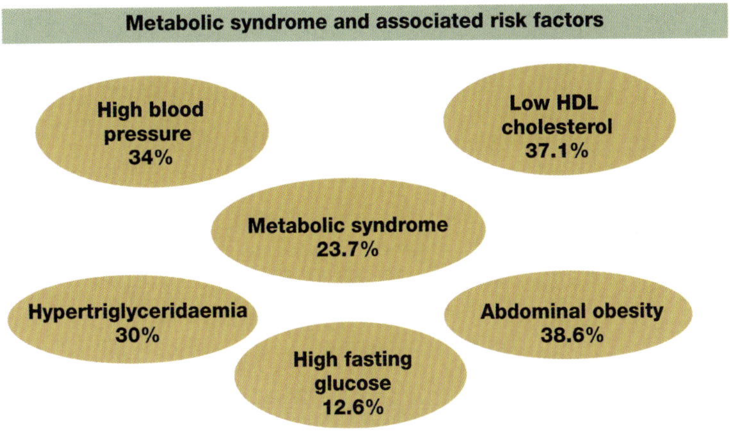

Fig 2.3 Demonstrates in the US adult population the prevalence of metabolic syndrome and its various correlates (adapted from Ford ES et al. *JAMA* 2002[28]).

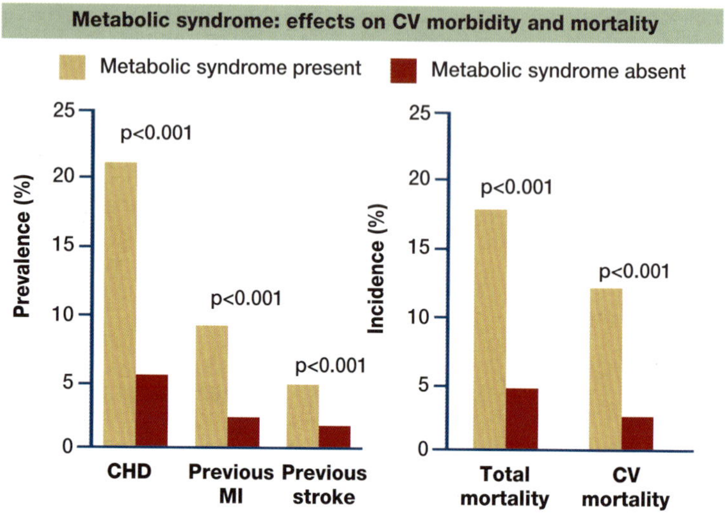

Fig 2.4 Effects of metabolic syndrome on morbidity and mortality from cardiovascular disease (adapted from Isomaa et al. *Diabetes Care* 2001;24:683-89 with permission from The American Diabetes Association).

Prevalence of obesity

Obesity is now a major public health issue, with increases in prevalence in UK adults from around 6% to 20% in men and 22% in women over the last few decades[27,33] (Fig 2.5). In the US around 30% of the adult population is clinically obese[34], although the rate of increase is now higher in the UK.

Definition of obesity

Obesity is normally defined as a body mass index >30 kg/m^2 and overweight as BMI >25 kg/m^2. Co-morbidities[35] start to increase significantly beyond BMI 27 kg/m^2.

Comorbidities include:

- cardiovascular disease
- hypertension
- dyslipidaemia
- type 2 diabetes
- certain types of cancer (gynaecological malignancy, prostate and bowel cancer).

Obesity has recently been redefined by WHO[36] in the Indo-Asian population as BMI >25 kg/m^2 and overweight as BMI >23 kg/m^2.

This is because people of Asian extraction tend to suffer the consequences of being overweight at lower levels of BMI, probably in part related to excess intra-abdominal fat accumulation and insulin resistance.

Evidence base for treatment of obesity

There is now hard evidence that significant weight loss, say around 10kg in an obese individual, is associated with dramatic risk reductions for morbidity and mortality (Table 2.1)[37]. In diabetic patients, even small degrees of weight loss are associated with clear health benefits and even weight maintenance (ie prevention of weight gain) is beneficial.

Standard 1 of the NSF for Diabetes discusses strategies for the prevention of the condition[13]. Several studies have now shown that programmes of mild caloric reduction in association with increased physical activity are associated with dramatic reductions in the risk of progression from impaired glucose to overt type 2 diabetes. Both the Diabetes Prevention Program[38] and the Finnish Diabetes Prevention Study[39] demonstrated risk reductions for progression from impaired glucose tolerance (IGT) to type 2 diabetes of almost 60% through lifestyle advice (Fig 2.6).

Prevalence of obesity in the UK

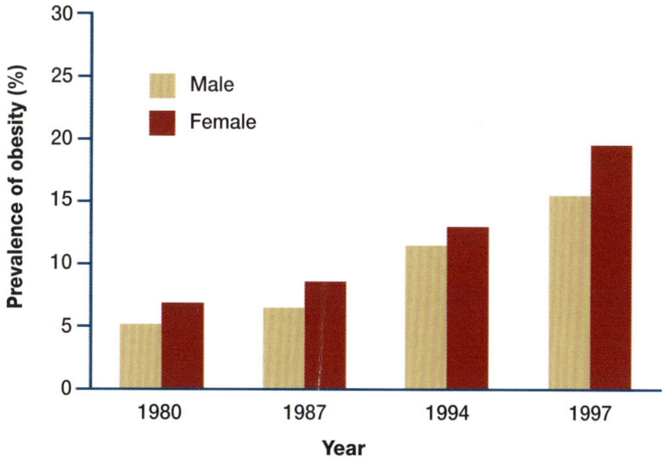

Fig 2.5 Demonstrates the dramatic increase in obesity rates in UK adults over the last few decades (adapted from British Nutrition Foundation 1999[27]).

Table 2.1: Consequences of weight loss of 10kg in an obese individual

Mortality ↓	Total = 20%	
	Diabetes related = 30%	
	Obesity related cancer = 40%	
Blood pressure ↓	Diastolic 20 mmHg	
	Systolic 10 mmHg	
Diabetes	↓ 50% fasting glucose	
Lipids	↓ Cholesterol	10%
	↓ LDL	15%
	↓ Triglycerides	30%
	↑ HDL	8%
	+ psychological and physical benefits	

(Adapted from Wilding and Williams, Blackwell Science, 1998[37])

More recently, the XENDOS (Xenical/Orlistat Prevention of Diabetes in Obese Subjects) trial[40] studied over 3,000 subjects with BMI >30kg/m^2. All were given a mildly hypocaloric diet and advised on moderate physical activity. They were randomised to receive the anti-obesity agent orlistat (an intestinal lipase inhibitor that prevents around 30% of fat absorption from the gut) or placebo. In the orlistat group there were significant reductions in risk for the development of type 2 diabetes, whether or not the patient had impaired glucose tolerance (Fig 2.7a, Fig 2.7b). Even the extra, rather modest, weight loss associated with orlistat treatment was associated with health benefits. The risk of developing diabetes was reduced by 37% in those treated with orlistat compared to those given lifestyle modifications alone. This is unlikely to be related to any special properties of orlistat beyond its anti-obesity effect: overall weight loss was 6.9kg in the orlistat group compared to 4.1kg in the diet/lifestyle only group over four years. It is important to note that not only was progression to type 2 diabetes reduced, but also other parameters of the metabolic syndrome were improved including reduction in LDL cholesterol and blood pressure compared with placebo.

Even in those with established diabetes, small degrees of weight loss are associated with increased survival times. Extrapolation suggests that a 10kg weight loss would restore around a third of the life expectancy in obese patients with type 2 diabetes[41].

The other anti-obesity agent currently available in the UK is sibutramine, which provides central appetite suppression[42]. This has also been associated with improvements in glycaemia in patients with diabetes. In addition it benefits other cardiovascular risk factors, including hypertension and dyslipidaemia. Sibutramine, however, should be used with caution in diabetic patients due to an occasional tendency to precipitate a significant rise in blood pressure.

Fig 2.6 Demonstrates dramatic risk reduction for progression from impaired glucose tolerance to type 2 diabetes through lifestyle advice, including weight loss and increased activity (adapted with permission from Diabetes Prevention Program Group, *New Engl J Med* 2002[38]).

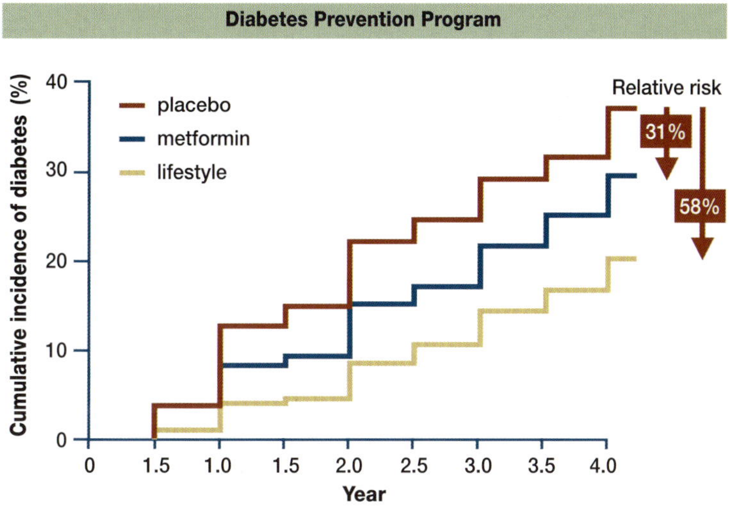

Fig 2.7a Demonstrates significant risk reduction in the development of type 2 diabetes (adapted from Torgerson JS et al. *Diabetes Care* 2004[40] with permission from The American Diabetes Association).

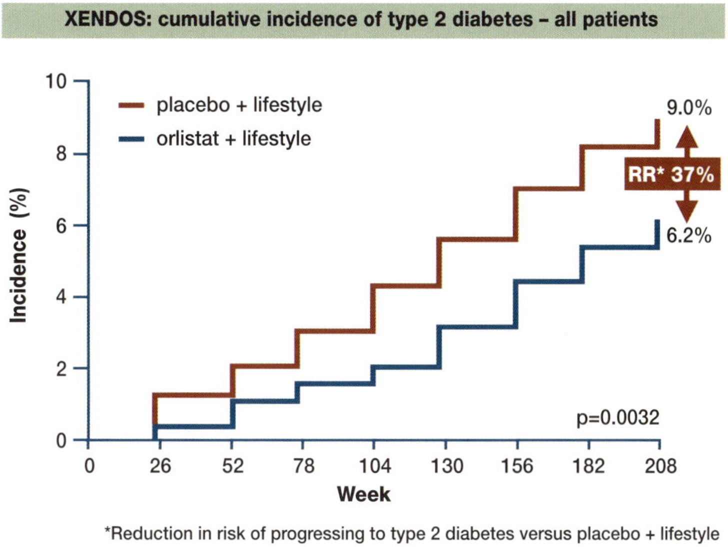

Fig 2.7b Diabetes in obese patients given the anti-obesity agent orlistat. Both groups had the same lifestyle advice regarding physical activity and dietary restriction (adapted from Torgerson JS et al. *Diabetes Care* 2004[40] with permission from the American Diabetes Association).

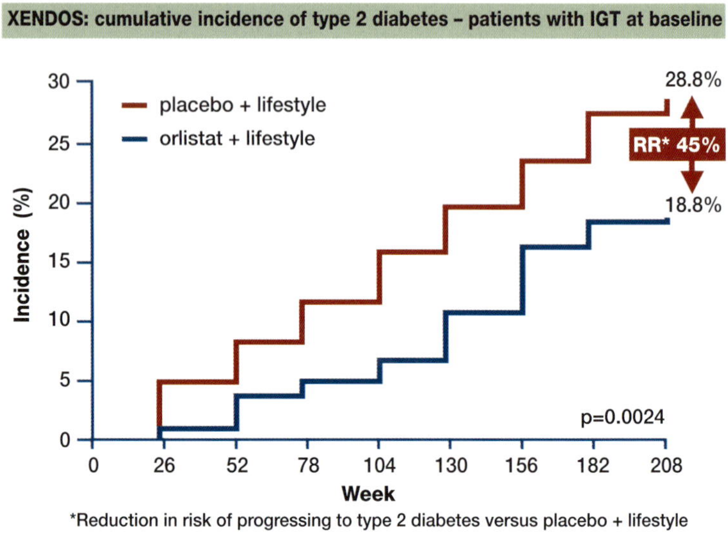

KEY LEARNING POINTS

Type 2 diabetes is part of the 'syndrome of chronic cardiovascular risk' and is commonly associated with dyslipidaemia and hypertension.

The co-occurrence of cardiovascular risk factors in the same patient relates to the primary underlying abnormality of insulin resistance, the main arbiters of which are obesity (particularly cental obesity) and reduced physical activity.

Obesity is a major health issue, affecting around 20% of men and 22% of women in the UK. Significant weight loss (10kg) is associated with dramatic risk reductions for mortality and morbidity.

3 Diabetes and dyslipidaemia

The typical dyslipidaemia of the metabolic/insulin resistance syndrome is reduced HDL cholesterol (the protective lipoprotein fraction) and increased triglycerides (↑LDL and VLDL)[26]. Diabetes is a pro-atherogenic state and characteristically patients also have increased levels of the high density, highly atherogenic LDL particles. Although mean LDL cholesterol is no higher in diabetic patients than in the general population, the actual atherogenic fraction is increased.

The reason for the development of these diabetes-related dyslipidaemias is not entirely clear but may relate in part to obesity. Studies have shown that production of VLDL is increased in obese patients[43]. This may relate to an increased turnover of non-esterified fatty acids stimulating the liver to produce more triglyceride-enriched VLDL, which results in increased triglycerides. The increase in VLDL leads to an increased exchange of VLDL triglycerides for cholesterol esters derived from HDL and LDL. This leads to a reduction in HDL cholesterol and formation of small dense atherogenic LDL particles.

It is also clear that for any given level of total or LDL cholesterol the risk is magnified in diabetic patients compared with the non-diabetic population[18]. The relationship between total cholesterol and coronary heart disease (CHD) risk is similar to that in the non-diabetic population in that it rises in parallel with increases in cholesterol, but the risk is increased four-fold compared with the non-diabetic population.

Evidence base for the management of dyslipidaemia

Until recently the evidence base for the treatment of diabetic dyslipidaemia relied entirely on extrapolation from studies in the general population. Indeed, a range of studies have clearly established for both primary and secondary prevention the value of lowering total and LDL cholesterol through the use of statins in the general population[11,44-48]. The basic message from these studies is that a 20% reduction in total serum cholesterol is associated with a relative risk reduction for coronary heart disease of around 30%. This is true for both men and women up to the age of 75 years. Some of these studies included diabetic patients[10,11]. However, it was only in the 4S Secondary Prevention Study that there was sufficient power for subgroup analysis to demonstrate similar benefits in diabetic patients[10].

The recently published Heart Protection Study[11] and the soon to be published Collaborative Atorvastatin Diabetes Study (CARDS) lays to rest any lingering doubts about the value of lowering lipids in diabetic patients. CARDS is the first study to specifically look at type 2 diabetic patients. Almost 3,000 patients from 132 sites in the UK and Ireland with type 2 diabetes, no prior coronary heart disease, but with at least one other risk factor were included. At entry, patients were required to have an LDL cholesterol ≤ 4.14mmol/l and triglycerides ≤ 6.78mmol/l. At randomisation, patients received either atorvastatin 10mg once daily or placebo with a minimum follow-up of four years. The primary endpoint was time to first major cardiac event (CHD, death, non-fatal myocardial infarction, re-vascularisation, unstable angina, stroke or resuscitated cardiac arrest)[49]. At the time of writing this study is about to report with apparently dramatic risk reductions for cardiovascular events and mortality in favour of atorvastatin.

The Heart Protection Study (HPS) with over 20,000 patients included almost 4,000 patients with diabetes, but without clinically evident cardiovascular disease. This study sought to determine the cholesterol lowering effects of simvastatin in patients at high risk of cardiovascular disease (ie they had had a previous cardiovascular event, or had diabetes or hypertension). The age range of the patients was up to 80 years and the lower limit for total cholesterol

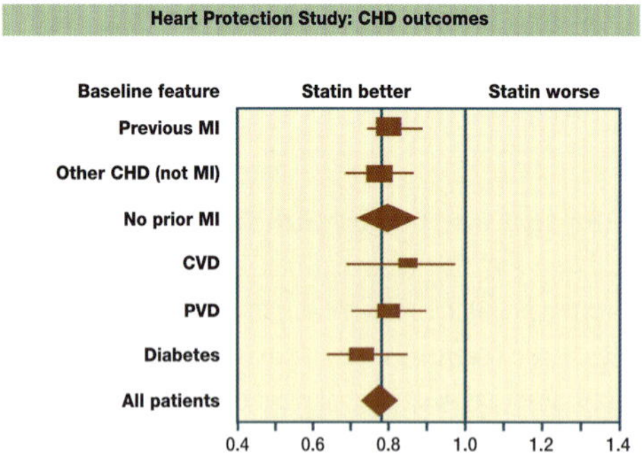

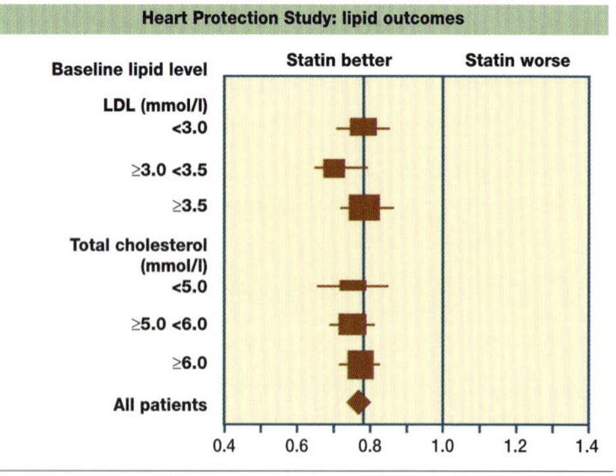

Fig 3.1a Demonstrates dramatic relative risk reduction for cardiovascular disease in both diabetic and non-diabetic subjects in the Heart Protection Study. **Fig 3.1b** Demonstrates the same relative risk reductions in the Heart Protection Study at all levels of serum cholesterol. (Adapted from Heart Protection Study Collaborative Group. *Lancet* 2002[11] with permission from Elsevier).

for entry into the trial was 3.5mmol/l. All patients received a fixed dose of 40mg simvastatin with no titration against serum cholesterol.

Over five years there was a relative risk reduction for coronary heart disease of approximately 30% in both the diabetic and non-diabetic subjects (Fig 3.1a). The same relative risk reduction was seen at all levels of serum cholesterol, with benefit up to 80 years (Fig 3.1b). There was also reduced risk not just for coronary heart disease, but for stroke, transient ischaemic attack and peripheral vascular disease (Fig 3.2).

The GREACE (GREek Atorvastatin and Coronary-heart-disease Evaluation) study[50] was designed to assess the long term survival of patients with coronary heart disease treated to the LDL cholesterol National Cholesterol Education Program (NCEP) target of <2.6 mmol/l. This is a much tighter target than previous studies. Sixteen hundred patients with established coronary heart disease and baseline LDL cholesterol >2.6 mmol/l with triglycerides <4.5 mmol/l had a mean follow-up of three years. They were randomised to receive atorvastatin 10-80 mg/day versus usual care. The primary endpoints included total mortality, coronary mortality and morbidity and stroke.

A mean atorvastatin dose of 24mg achieved less than 2.6mmol/l for LDL target in 95% of patients versus 3% of the usual care group. Treating to target of <2.6mmol/l for LDL cholesterol reduced cardiovascular events by half! (Fig 3.3). The statin was extremely well tolerated and cost effective.

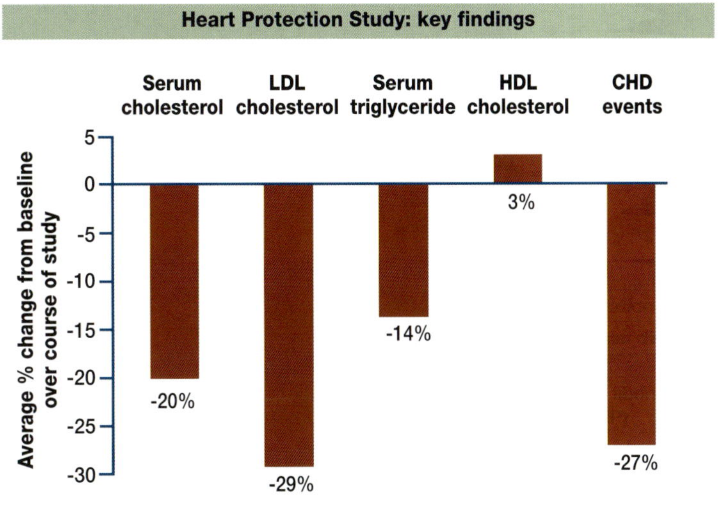

Fig 3.2 Demonstrates similar and dramatic risk reductions for all cardiovascular events and specifically for diabetic patients with statin treatment (adapted from Heart Protection Study Collaborative Group. *Lancet* 2002[11] with permission from Elsevier).

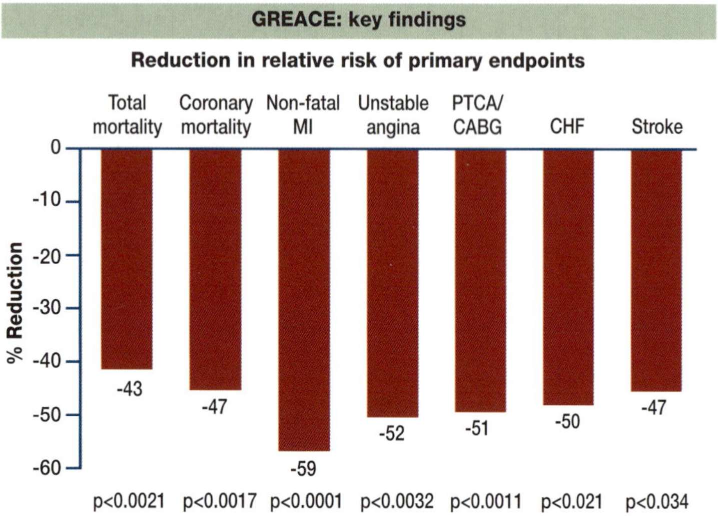

Fig 3.3 Demonstrates relative risk reduction for primary endpoints compared with usual treatment groups (adapted from Athyros VG et al. *Curr Med Res Opin* 2002[50]).

A diabetes substudy of GREACE has also recently reported[51]. This included 313 patients with diabetes who had a history of myocardial infarction or >70% coronary stenosis. Baseline LDL was >2.6mmol/l, triglycerides <4.5mmol/l and mean follow-up was three years. Patients were randomised to receive atorvastatin or 'usual care'. The primary endpoints were identical to those previously described. At baseline mean total cholesterol was 7mmol/l, LDL cholesterol 4.9mmol/l, HDL 0.9mmol/l and triglycerides 2.5mmol/l.

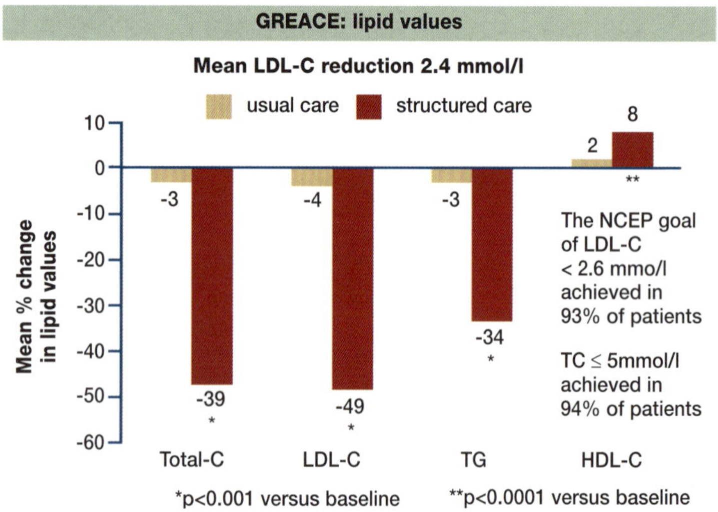

Fig 3.4 Demonstrates mean percentage change in lipid values (adapted from Athyros VG et al. *Angiology*, 2003[51] with permission from Westminster Publications).

Using atorvastatin, the LDL-C goal of <2.6 mmol/l was achieved in 93% of patients in the active group (Fig 3.4). There were dramatic reductions in three-year mortality and morbidity rates in favour of the atorvastatin group (Fig 3.5 and Fig 3.6).

Fig 3.5 Demonstrates three-year mortality and morbidity rates (adapted from Athyros VG et al. *Angiology*, 2003[51] with permission from Westminster Publications).

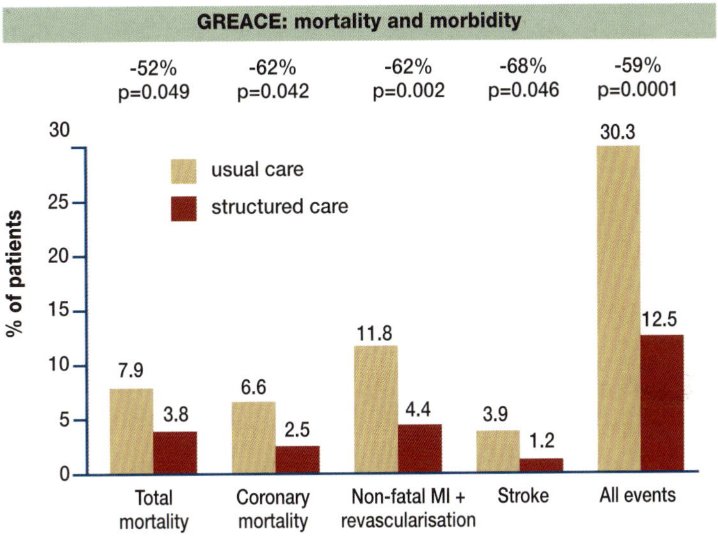

Fig 3.6 Demonstrates event rate for all events in the GREACE study (adapted from Athyros VG et al. *Angiology*, 2003[51] with permission from Westminster Publications).

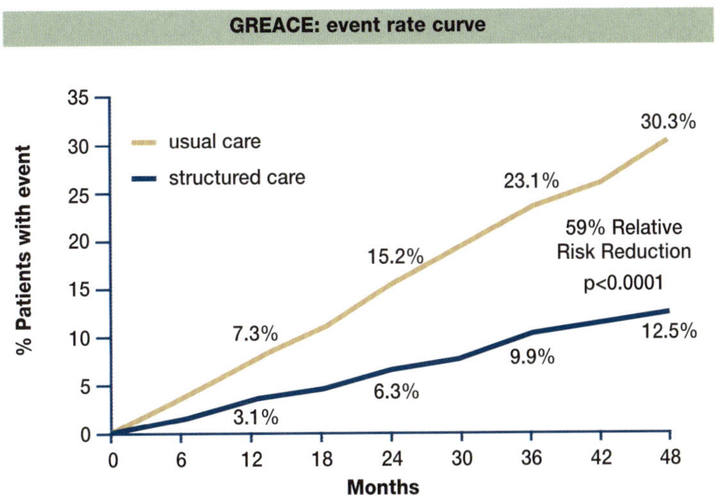

The recent Anglo-Scandinavian Cardiac Outcomes Trial – lipid lowering arm (ASCOT-LLA)[52] looked at the benefits of cholesterol lowering in the primary prevention of coronary heart disease in hypertensive patients who were not significantly dyslipidaemic. Around 20,000 patients were randomly assigned to additional atorvastatin 10mg or placebo. The planned follow-up was for five years and the primary endpoint was non-fatal myocardial infarction and fatal coronary heart disease. The treatment was stopped early after a median follow-up of 3.3 years due to the significant reduction in primary events in the statin group compared to placebo (relative risk reduction=36%) with a lowering of total serum cholesterol of 1.1mmol/l after three years of follow-up.

In addition, three-year sub-group analysis of around 2,500 hypertensive patients with type 2 diabetes and raised cholesterol demonstrated a 23% reduction in total cardiovascular events.

It is clear that, based on this work and other studies, LDL cholesterol targets will come down and to achieve this the more powerful statins will commonly be necessary.

The authors therefore believe that the concept of primary prevention in type 2 diabetes is redundant and that statin therapy intervention should not be determined by levels of serum cholesterol alone. In the HPS, patients all showed similar relative risk reductions whatever the baseline level of cholesterol. This has to some extent been recognised by the recent NICE guidance, which recommends that diabetic patients with a 10-year CHD risk >15% should receive a statin whatever the level of baseline cholesterol[12]. In practice, this means that around 70% of all patients with type 2 diabetes should be given a statin. For those patients who do not meet the >15% 10-year CHD risk requirement, this is normally because of their relative youth. Thus the question that needs to be asked is why should it be necessary to wait 10 years for a 35-year-old type 2 diabetic patient to reach age 45 so as to enter into the 15% 10-year CHD risk range before statin treatment can be recommended. The only reason for withholding statin treatment in this case is age, leaving the patient with the potential for progressive development of atherosclerosis over 10 years. It is the opinion of the authors that all adult patients with type 2 diabetes should be offered statin therapy.

Management of dyslipidaemia in diabetic patients

Lifestyle advice including the importance of regular exercise and weight management is an important part of therapy. The evidence base for statins is, however, now so strong that these agents should normally be given to all patients with type 2 diabetes unless there is a major contraindication or tolerability problem. This probably also applies to all adult patients with type 1 diabetes, although care should be taken in women of reproductive age as statins should not be used in the peri-conception period, during pregnancy or during breast feeding.

HMG-CoA reductase inhibitors (statins)

These agents have been associated with profound reductions in cardiovascular risk and mortality. The evidence points to the degree of lowering of LDL cholesterol as the major reason for this, although there is interesting data showing these agents may also reduce inflammation, which could relate to risk reduction[53]. They are competitive inhibitors of HMG-CoA reductase[53], the enzyme involved in the rate-limiting step in cholesterol biosynthesis through conversion of HMG-CoA to mevalonate. They act by reducing hepatic cholesterol synthesis with up-regulation of LDL receptors and a fall in plasma LDL concentrations.

Statins can cause a reduction in LDL of up to 40% with maximum effect if the drug is given at bedtime as most hepatic cholesterol biosynthesis occurs overnight. The tolerability profile is good, although it is recommended that liver function tests and plasma creatinine kinase levels are measured before starting therapy and intermittently thereafter. Although cerivastatin has been withdrawn because of increased risks of rhabdomyolysis the other agents (atorvastatin, fluvastatin, pravastatin and simvastatin) appear much safer.

The evidence we have for LDL cholesterol is: *the lower, the better*. This emphasises that the more powerful statins such as atorvastatin or simvastatin should normally be the statin of choice.

Rosuvastatin is the newest statin on the market and has a higher potency than traditional statins[53]. It has been shown to significantly reduce LDL cholesterol and at the same time raise HDL cholesterol and lower triglycerides[54]. It lacks the evidence base associated with the more traditional agents, but despite this, the Clinical Trials Programme[55-57] has demonstrated profound reductions in LDL cholesterol, with target levels reached in the majority of patients, even at the lowest doses.

Cholesterol absorption inhibitors

The first of these, ezetimibe, has recently appeared on the market[58]. These agents are particularly useful in combination with statins where LDL cholesterol targets are not being met. They provide an extra, approximately 18% reduction in LDL cholesterol acting by a different mechanism (through reduction in cholesterol absorption) rather than (as statins do) liver synthesis[58,59]. They are also useful where statins are not tolerated or contraindicated. Not only is LDL cholesterol reduced, but there is also evidence for small increases in HDL cholesterol and a reduction in triglycerides compared with placebo[58-61]. The tolerability and safety profiles appear excellent.

As there is now a hard evidence base for statin usage in reducing cardiovascular morbidity and mortality, these new agents will mainly be used in combination. This allows for lower doses of statins to be used thereby reducing the risks of side effects and may also have a role in patients who cannot tolerate statins and in situations where powerful drug effects in combination with high-dose statins are needed such as in patients with familial hypercholesterolaemia.

These agents may also be useful for co-administration with a fibrate. Although this combination is not licensed at present, it might be particularly relevant in type 2 diabetes, where the common lipid related problems include raised triglycerides, low HDL and increases in the small dense atherogenic LDL.

Fibrates

The typical dyslipidaemia of type 2 diabetes of low HDL and raised triglycerides would suggest a significant role for fibrates and there is some evidence supporting this[62]. If the patient has a normal total cholesterol with <15% 10-year CHD risk, low HDL and raised triglycerides then it could be argued that fibrates should be given as first-line treatment. More commonly, a statin would be the first-line treatment, bringing in a fibrate combination if the HDL remains low with raised triglycerides. This combination may be associated with an increased risk of side effects and more careful monitoring may be required.

KEY LEARNING POINTS
Patients with diabetes typically have ↓HDL cholesterol and ↑LDL and ↑VLDL
A 20% reduction in serum cholesterol is associated with a relative risk reduction for coronary heart disease of around 30%
All patients with type 2 diabetes should be offered statin therapy unless there is a major contraindication or tolerability problem
Cholesterol absorption inhibitors can be used in combination with statins and may have a role to play in patients who cannot tolerate statins
It is the authors' opinion that all patients with type 2 diabetes should be on a statin so that when fibrates are indicated, this would normally be in combination

4 Diabetes and hypertension

Definition of hypertension

Type 2 diabetes is part of a syndrome of chronic cardiovascular risk and commonly co-associated with dyslipidaemia and hypertension. The old WHO criteria defined hypertension as a blood pressure of 160/95mmHg or greater and on this basis around half of all patients with type 2 diabetes can be classified as hypertensive. Applying the newer, more strict, criteria (eg British Hypertension Society definition of hypertension as blood pressure ≥ 140/90mmHg[15]) around 80% of diabetics would be included. Why hypertension should be so prevalent in type 2 diabetes is not entirely clear but presumably relates to insulin resistance, possibly the effects of hyperinsulinaemia and the increased tendency to retain sodium by the kidneys and increased sympathetic nervous system stimulation[26]. Obesity is a major risk factor for hypertension and this is particularly marked in association with central adiposity, which in turn strongly relates to insulin resistance and cardiovascular risk.

Evidence base for the management of hypertension

The evidence base for the benefits of blood pressure lowering in diabetic patients was, until five years ago, extrapolated from results in the general population. In 1998 the United Kingdom Prospective Diabetes Study (UKPDS) reported showing the clear benefits not just of improved glycaemic control[7], but also of tight blood pressure treatment[8] (Table 4.1). Patients were randomised into tight and conventional blood pressure groups with separation over the nine years of the study of around 10mmHg systolic and 5mmHg diastolic in favour of tight blood pressure control. This was associated with dramatic risk reductions for microvascular endpoints (retinopathy and nephropathy), diabetes-related endpoints, death related to diabetes and stroke.

Since then a range of studies have reported on the benefits of blood pressure lowering in diabetic patients. In the Hypertension Optimal Treatment (HOT) study almost 20,000 patients aged from 50 to 80 years, with mild to moderate diastolic hypertension (100-115mmHg), were randomised to target diastolic blood pressures of <80, 85 or 90mmHg respectively[9]. The benefits of blood pressure

Table 4.1: UKPDS data showing vascular risk reductions consequent on tight glycaemic and blood pressure control[7,8]

Glycaemic control: tight versus conventional (HbA_{1c} 7% versus 7.9%)

Endpoint	Relative Risk ↓ (%)	p
Microvascular	25	0.010
Myocardial infarction	16	0.052
Diabetes-related	12	0.029

Blood pressure: tight versus conventional (144/82 versus 154/87mmHg)

Endpoint	Relative Risk ↓ (%)	p
Microvascular	37	0.010
Diabetes-related	24	0.005
Deaths related to diabetes	32	0.020
Stroke	44	0.013

reduction were particularly profound in the large group of patients with diabetes. These patients showed around 50% reduction in major cardiovascular events where the target blood pressure was <80mmHg compared to those where the target pressure was <90mmHg (Fig 4.1). The HOT study also demonstrated the benefits of low-dose aspirin (75mg) with around 15% reduction in cardiovascular endpoints and mortality (but at the expense of increased risk of non-fatal haemorrhagic episodes).

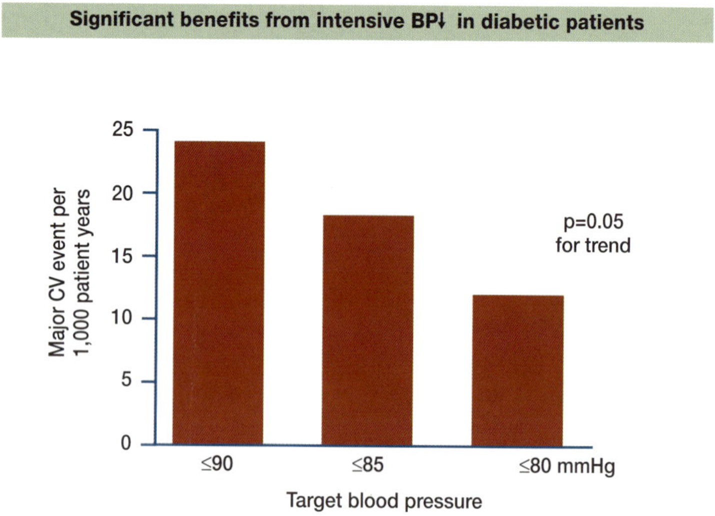

Fig 4.1
Demonstrates the halving of major cardiovascular event rates in diabetic patients in the group assigned to tightest blood pressure control compared with those with more relaxed control (adapted from Hansson L, et al. *Lancet* 1998[9] with permission from Elsevier).

Fig 4.2
Demonstrates the overall risk reduction in the primary composite endpoint of myocardial infarction, stroke or death in the HOPE study (adapted from HOPE Study Investigators. *Lancet* 2000[66] with permission from Elsevier).

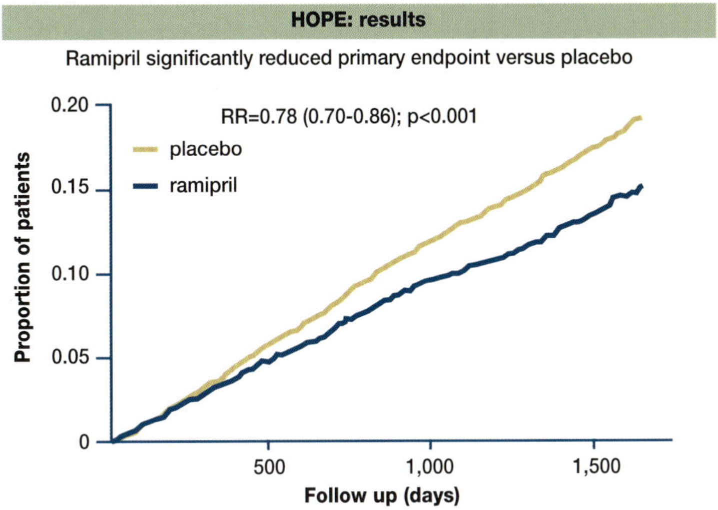

In all, six large randomised prospective trials have now shown the profound benefits of antihypertensive treatment on cardiovascular morbidity and mortality in diabetic patients. The other four included the Systolic Hypertension in the Elderly Programme (SHEP)[63], Systolic Hypertension in Europe (SYST-EUR) trial (calcium channel blocker based therapy)[64], Captopril Prevention Project (CAPPP)[65] and the Heart Outcomes Prevention Evaluation (HOPE) study[66] (Fig 4.2, Fig 4.3) (both of the latter studies were

Fig 4.3
Demonstrates individual cardiovascular outcome in the HOPE study (adapted from HOPE Study Investigators. *Lancet* 2000[66] with permission from Elsevier).

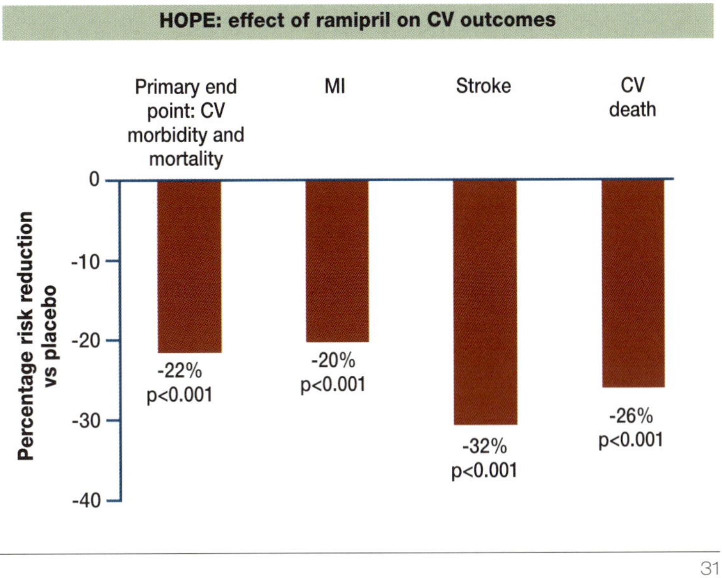

ACE inhibitor based). All showed significant reductions in cardiovascular event rates and mortality, the latter two compared with standard antihypertensive treatments.

All of these studies emphasised that one of the most cost-effective and beneficial things that clinicians can do for diabetic patients is to aggressively manage their blood pressure.

Management of hypertension in diabetes

Non-pharmacological strategies (Box 4.1) may be of significant benefit in reducing blood pressure, but the majority of patients will require at least one antihypertensive or multiple antihypertensive therapies to get down to target. Drug therapy should not be too long delayed and never in those with evidence of end-organ damage or at high cardiovascular risk (>15% over 10 years).

Box 4.1: Non-pharmacological measures

Patients should be advised on:

- weight loss where appropriate
- not adding salt to food
- increased physical activity
- reduction of alcohol intake
- cessation of cigarette smoking

Blood pressure control in the diabetic patient, although essential, may be difficult. The ideal antihypertensive agent for a diabetic patient should:

- lower blood pressure effectively
- have an excellent tolerability profile
- have metabolic neutrality
- have the ability to combine with any other antihypertensive agent
- have evidence for cardiac and renal protection
- avoid increasing the risk of erectile dysfunction (very common in male patients with diabetes), impairment of limb blood flow and postural hypotension.

Table 4.2 shows the range of antihypertensive classes available. All are useful in diabetic patients and since most will require combination treatment, it is extremely useful to have a range of different antihypertensives from which to choose. The main message is: *Get the blood pressure down and keep it down by whatever means*; this is more relevant than which drugs should be used as first-line or second-line therapy. However, certain classes of antihypertensive agents may be preferred as first- or second-line compared to others.

Table 4.2: The different classes of antihypertensives

	Thiazides	β-blockers	Calcium channel blockers	α-blockers	ACE inhibitors	ARBs
Glycaemia	↑	↑	–	–	–	–
Lipids	↑	↑	–	–	(↓)	(↓)
Electrolytes	K^+ reduction	–	–	–	-	-
Insulin resistance	↑	↑	–	–	(↓)	(↓)
Erectile dysfunction	↑	↑	–	–	–	–

↑ deterioration (↓) = possible improvement – neutral effect

Note the work on thiazides showing metabolic deterioration was done with high-dose thiazides. Low-dose thiazides have equal blood pressure lowering effects with reduced risk of metabolic side effects. Indapamide is a thiazide-like diuretic that appears to be metabolically neutral. The deleterious effects of β-blockers have probably also been overstated. Combination treatment with antihypertensives from different classes is normally required to get down to blood pressure targets.

Thiazides

These drugs are inexpensive, have been around a long time and have well-known safety profiles[67]. They can normally be given once daily, but their use may be associated with metabolic deterioration in diabetic patients from the point of view of glycaemia and lipids. They can also provoke hypokalaemia and erectile dysfunction. It should, however, be emphasised that most of the studies in this area were done many years ago with high-dose diuretics. In fact these drugs will give the same level of blood pressure reduction at lower doses, reducing the risk of side effects. Furthermore, trials have demonstrated cardiovascular protection with a reduction in the incidence of stroke, heart failure and risk of cardiovascular disease.

Thiazide-like diuretics such as indapamide, which is now also available in a slow-release form, may be of particular interest[68-71]. The mechanism of action includes a reduction in arteriole and total peripheral resistance with improved arterial compliance and a diuretic effect on the kidney. This agent appears to have metabolic neutrality in a slow-release formulation and a 24-hour antihypertensive profile.

Studies have demonstrated reduced left ventricular hypertrophy, which appears in part independent of blood pressure lowering with possibly a direct and progressive effect on the heart. It has also been shown to be associated with a reduction in protein excretion for patients with type 2 diabetes and microalbuminuria[72,73].

Fig 4.4 Demonstrates relative risk reduction for stroke of 28% and major vascular events of 25% in the PROGRESS study (adapted from PROGRESS Collaborative Group. *Lancet* 2001[74] with permission from Elsevier).

Results from the PROGRESS study

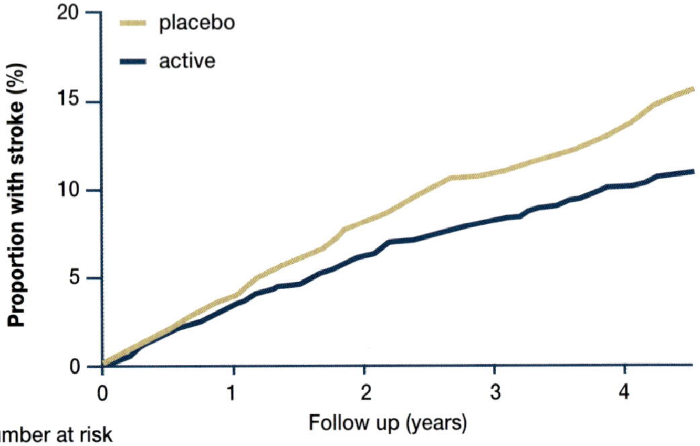

Number at risk

	0	1	2	3	4
Active	3,051	2,902	2,765	2,634	1,595
Placebo	3,054	2,880	2,707	2,551	1,533

A recent study (PROGRESS) included 6,000 patients with a previous history of stroke or transient ischaemic attack. Patients were randomised to receive the ACE inhibitor, perindopril, or placebo[74]. Indapamide and perindopril combination therapy could be used in the active group. Patients were either hypertensive or normotensive and were followed for four years. There was a relative risk reduction for stroke of 28% and major vascular events of 25% (Fig 4.4). This improvement was particularly apparent in patients receiving combination therapy with an overall stroke risk reduction of 43%, irrespective of whether the patient was hypertensive or normotensive.

The recent ALLHAT study (Antihypertensive and Lipid Lowering treatment to prevent Heart Attack Trial) also extolled the benefits of chlortalidone, another thiazide-like diuretic[75]. This was a very large study where the objective was to determine whether treatment with a calcium channel blocker or an ACE inhibitor lowered the incidence of cardiovascular events compared with treatment using a thiazide. The primary outcome was combined fatal coronary heart disease or non-fatal myocardial infarction. Over approximately five years, there was no difference between the treatments for the primary outcome. In addition, all-cause mortality did not differ between the groups. It can be concluded from this trial that thiazide-type diuretics are at least as good as ACE inhibitors or calcium channel blockers for the management of hypertension. These agents can now be used as first-line therapy for the management of hypertension in diabetes. It was noted, however, that ALLHAT non-diabetic patients in the thiazide group had a higher rate of progression to type 2 diabetes compared with the other groups.

Beta-blockers

These agents are relatively inexpensive and effective in lowering blood pressure, with evidence for cardiovascular protection, particularly after myocardial infarction[67]. The UKPDS hypertension arm demonstrated that use of the beta-blocker, atenolol, was associated with reduced cardiovascular risk and mortality in patients with type 2 diabetes[8].

Negative issues include poor tolerability and a high rate of side effects including metabolic disturbance, erectile dysfunction and a reduction in warning symptoms of hypoglycaemia[67]. (The latter is almost certainly over-estimated and not usually a problem.)

These drugs are particularly useful where there is co-incident hypertension and angina. Otherwise, the authors would not normally recommend beta-blockers as first-line treatment for hypertension in diabetes.

Calcium channel blockers

The non-dihydropyridine calcium channel blockers such as amlodipine or felodipine are suitable for once daily dosing and are the agents within this class that are normally recommended for hypertension treatment. They are relatively inexpensive, efficacious in lowering blood pressure and have peripheral vasodilating properties; they also have the added advantage of being antianginal, antiarrhythmic and cardioprotective. These agents are metabolically neutral and there is evidence for improved coronary blood flow and regression of left ventricular hypertrophy[67].

Calcium channel blockers have a relatively good safety profile, but there is a high incidence of minor side effects such as facial flushing and ankle oedema[67]. They can be used as first-line agents for the management of hypertension in diabetes, although the authors prefer to use alternative agents first line.

Specific alpha-blockers

Doxazosin is the only specific alpha-blocker currently in use in the UK. The old alpha-blockers are also still available such as prazosin, but have tended to have a high incidence of side effects, particularly first-dose hypotension and postural hypotension[67].

These agents are efficacious in lowering blood pressure, although there is no hard outcome data that would support their use as first-line therapy. They were studied in the ALLHAT trial[75], but interim analysis reported a 25% increase in risk of combined cardiovascular endpoints compared to thiazides. The doxazosin group was discontinued. The problems mainly related to heart failure (although the definition used remains controversial) and stroke, but there was no evidence of increased mortality.

They are metabolically neutral and are useful in combination, but should not normally be used as first-line agents.

Angiotensin converting enzyme (ACE) inhibitors

These agents inhibit the renin angiotensin system (RAS), which itself is profoundly implicated in the maintenance of blood pressure and development of hypertension[67]. ACE inhibitors inhibit the angiotensin converting enzyme, which is involved in the conversion of inactive angiotensin I to active angiotensin II (Fig 4.5)[76].

These agents:

- are effective in lowering blood pressure
- are metabolically neutral
- have a good side effect profile
- reverse left ventricular hypertrophy

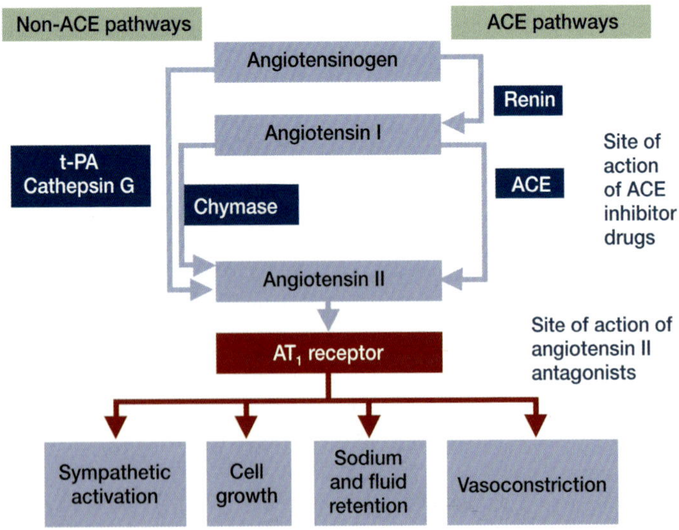

Fig 4.5 Demonstrates the renin angiotensin system and the site of action of ACE inhibitors and angiotensin II receptor blockers (adapted from Thompson Publishing Services. In: *Clinical Management of Hypertension*. Barnett AH (ed). London: Martin Dunitz. 2002;52).

- have an excellent evidence base for treatment in patients with congestive heart failure, with reduction in morbidity and mortality[67].

There is also a suggestion in non-diabetic patients that ACE inhibitors reduce the risk of developing type 2 diabetes. They have been shown to decrease elevated systemic vascular resistance, reduce sympathetic tone and enhance perfusion of the heart and kidneys. There is also evidence that they are reno- and cardioprotective.

The HOPE study demonstrated cardiovascular protection, which appeared to be over and above the effects of systemic blood pressure lowering[66]. Some 3,500 of the 9,500 patients studied had diabetes and these had a history of cardiovascular disease or at least one other cardiovascular risk factor. The aim of the study was to examine the incidence of cardiovascular endpoints and mortality and patients were randomised to either ACE inhibition (ramipril) or placebo. This trial did not aim to compare blood pressure lowering effects in that both groups had the same blood pressure targets and other anti-hypertensives could be used.

The five-year study was terminated a year early because of the profound cardiovascular and mortality benefits shown in favour of ACE inhibition (see Fig 4.2 and Fig 4.3). This was apparent from 6-8 months after randomisation.

Two further studies support the cardiovascular protective properties of ACE inhibitors[65,74]. The CAPPP study was a six-year, randomised trial that compared ACE inhibition with captopril against a beta-blocker or thiazide. In the 600 diabetic patients there was no significant difference in blood pressure, but the ACE inhibitor group showed significant reductions in myocardial infarction of 34% and cardiac events of 67%[65].

This data gained support from the PROGRESS study (see Fig 4.4)[74]. ACE inhibition with perindopril, with or without indapamide, was compared with placebo in patients who previously had had a cerebrovascular accident or transient ischaemic attack. This was associated with a relative risk reduction for stroke of 28% and for total major vascular events of 25%. The combination of ACE inhibitor and indapamide was associated with a stroke risk reduction of 43%. These findings were not related to whether the patient was hypertensive or normotensive.

ACE inhibitors have also been shown to have benefit in combination with diuretics in heart failure. This is because of a reduction in cardiovascular morbidity and mortality[67].

The main concern with ACE inhibitors is the development of a chronic cough, which may result in discontinuation in around 1-in-10 patients. First-dose hypotension is reported, but rare. For this reason ACE inhibitors should be started at the lowest doses and titrated to the highest evidence-base dose over several weeks. Discontinuation of diuretics for a few days before and just after starting an ACE inhibitor may also reduce these risks, although in most cases this is unnecessary. A major contraindication to ACE inhibition is the presence of renal artery stenosis because of possible deterioration of renal function. This is an extremely rare occurrence, but it is still recommended to check creatinine 7-10 days after starting an ACE inhibitor and after each dose increment.

In conclusion, these agents should be considered as suitable first-line treatments for the management of hypertension in diabetes because of their efficacy, excellent side-effect profile, ability to combine with any other antihypertensive class, metabolic neutrality and evidence for cardiac and renal protection.

Angiotensin II receptor blockers (ARBs)

These agents also inhibit the renin angiotensin system, but through a direct blocking effect of the angiotensin II receptor (see Fig 4.5)[67,76]. They are efficacious in lowering blood pressure, have probably the best side-effect profile of all antihypertensives, are less likely to cause chronic cough than ACE inhibitors and are metabolically neutral.

Until recently, the evidence base has not been sufficient to support their use for first-line therapy, but there is now evidence demonstrating both cardiac and renal protection and that these agents may be useful in heart failure.

Three studies have looked at renal protection in some detail in hypertensive patients with type 2 diabetes. Two of these studies were part of the PRIME programme using the angiotensin II receptor blocker, irbesartan, to study prevention of diabetic nephropathy[77] and also reduction in progression of established diabetic nephropathy[78].

The first of these studies (IRMA2) involved almost 600 hypertensive type 2 diabetic patients with microalbuminuria[77]. They were randomised to once daily therapy with low-dose irbesartan (150mg), high-dose irbesartan (300mg) or placebo. In addition, other antihypertensive agents could be added and the blood pressure goal was identical in all three groups (<135/85mmHg). The primary endpoint was time to onset of overt diabetic nephropathy defined as an albumin excretion rate >200 μg/min and an increase of at least 30% from baseline.

The high-dose irbesartan group was associated with a relative risk reduction of 70% for progression to overt diabetic nephropathy compared to the control group ($p<0.001$) (Fig 4.6a and Fig 4.6b). The relative risk reduction for the low-dose irbesartan group was almost 40%, but this did not reach significance ($p=0.08$). Using 'numbers needed to treat' analysis, it is calculated that it would be necessary to treat 10 patients with irbesartan 300mg once daily for two years to prevent one patient from progressing from microalbuminuria to overt diabetic nephropathy. This appears to be highly cost effective.

The second report (IDNT) was of a study of around 1,700 hypertensive type 2 diabetic patients[78]. The aim of this three-year trial was to compare the effects of irbesartan with placebo and the calcium channel blocker, amlodipine. The blood pressure goals were the same in all three groups (<135/85mmHg) and other drugs could be added to treat blood pressure. At randomisation patients could have a normal or raised creatinine, but required significant proteinuria. The primary outcome was time to a composite endpoint of doubling of the baseline creatinine level, end-stage renal disease and death. For the primary endpoint the irbesartan group showed a relative risk reduction of 20% compared to placebo ($p=0.02$) and 23% compared to amlodipine ($p=0.006$) (Fig 4.7).

IRMA 2: Primary endpoint

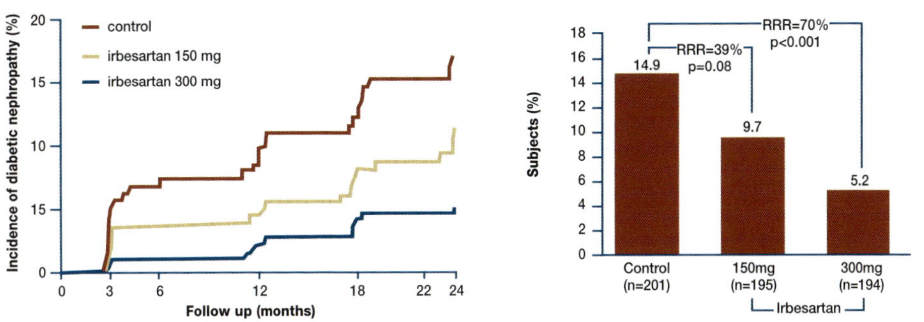

Fig 4.6a and Fig 4.6b Demonstrate the relative risk reduction of 70% for progression to overt diabetic nephropathy compared to placebo in the IRMA2 study (Fig 4.6a adapted with permission from Parving H-H, et al. *N Engl J Med* 2001[77]).

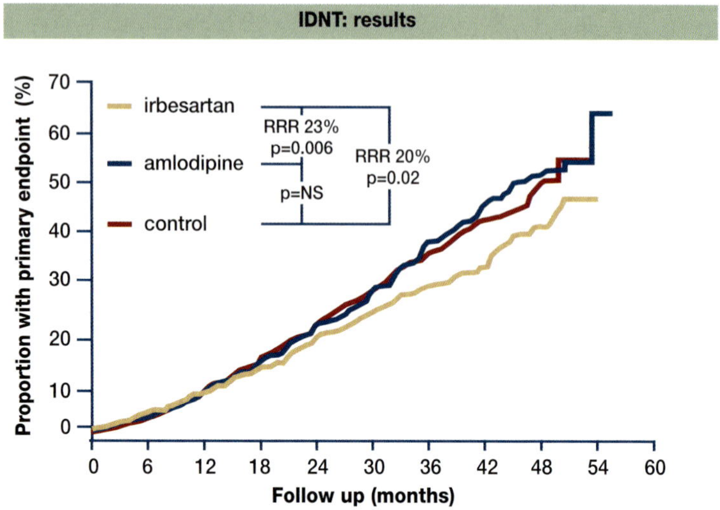

Fig 4.7 Demonstrates a 20% reduction compared to placebo and 23% compared to amlodipine for the angiotensin II receptor blocker irbesartan in the IDNT study for the primary endpoint which was a composite of doubling of the baseline creatinine level, end stage renal disease and death (adapted with permission from Lewis EJ, et al. *N Engl J Med* 2001[78]).

Extrapolation from these results suggest that by treating 15 hypertensive patients with significant proteinuria for three years with irbesartan, one patient would be saved from doubling of baseline creatinine level, development of end-stage renal disease or death – again highly cost effective.

A further study in overt diabetic nephropathy (RENAAL) compared the angiotensin II receptor blocker, losartan with placebo in hypertensive type 2 diabetic patients with proteinuria. The relative risk reduction for the primary composite endpoint (similar to that in IDNT) was 16% compared to the control group ($p=0.02$)[79].

From the point of view of cardiovascular protection, the Losartan Intervention For the Endpoint reduction in hypertension (LIFE) trial compared losartan with atenolol in patients with left ventricular hypertrophy[80]. The primary composite endpoint (cardiovascular mortality, fatal/non-fatal stroke, fatal/non-fatal myocardial infarction) was reduced by almost 15% ($p<0.009$) in the ARB group compared to the beta-blocker group.

The Candesartan in Heart failure Assessment of Reduction in Mortality and morbidity (CHARM) programme is the largest trial ever undertaken in patients with heart failure. Comparison used the angiotensin receptor blocker candesartan versus placebo in three different populations with class 2–4 heart failure[81-84].

Three different studies were conducted:

- **CHARM-added**: randomised around 2,500 patients with

ejection fractions of approximately ≤ 40% treated with optimum doses of ACE inhibitors

- **CHARM-alternative**: randomised around 2,000 patients with ejection fractions ≤ 40% who were intolerant of ACE inhibitors
- **CHARM-preserved**: randomised around 3,000 patients with ejection fractions >40%.

The trials were combined for analysis into the CHARM-overall programme. After pre-specified analysis using covariant adjustment, there was a statistically significant reduction in the primary endpoint of mortality (hazard ratio) of 0.09 (ie 10%, with confidence limits between 0.82 and 0.94, p=0.032). There was a highly significant absolute reduction in the combined incidence of cardiovascular death and hospitalisation for heart failure of around 16% (p=0.0001) with a reduction in the number of patients developing diabetes of 6% versus 7.4%, (p=0.02) (Fig 4.8).

The consistency in the results led to an editorial in *The Lancet* which stated that over three years the treatment effect would equate to one death prevented per 63 patients treated, one first hospitalisation with heart failure prevented per 23 patients treated, and one new case of diabetes prevented per 71 patients treated[85].

The conclusion is that ARBs should be prescribed in addition to ACE inhibitors, beta-blockers and/or spironolactone in patients with ejection fractions <40% and as an alternative to ACE

Fig 4.8 Effect of candesartan on cardiovascular mortality or hospital admission for congestive heart failure (CHARM programme) (adapted from Pfeffer MA, et al. *Lancet* 2003[81] with permission from Elsevier).

CHARM: results

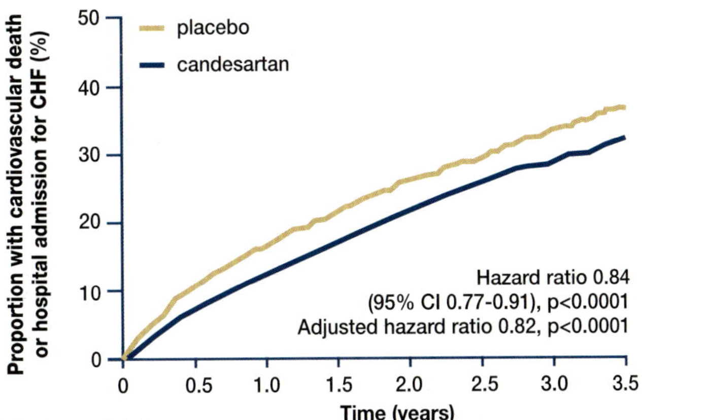

Numbers at risk

Candesartan	3,803	3,563	3,271	2,215	761
Placebo	3,796	3,464	3,170	2,157	743

inhibitors in patients with ACE inhibitor intolerance. These agents can also be used in patients with ejection fractions >40% to reduce risk of hospitalisation with heart failure.

Angiotensin II receptor blockers can now be considered suitable as first-line agents for the management of hypertension in diabetes, particularly where there is evidence of micro- or macro-proteinuria. They also show cardioprotective properties including in cases of heart failure. They have an excellent side-effect profile and can be combined with any other antihypertensive class with good evidence for renal protection and increasing evidence for cardiac protection. They can also be given once daily and there is some evidence in the elderly that they are particularly beneficial for systolic hypertension.

Combination treatment

Since the primary objective is to get the blood pressure down and keep it down, long term, it is necessary to use all classes of antihypertensive agents in order to choose the right combination for the individual patient. The great majority of hypertensive diabetic patients will require multiple antihypertensive therapies in combination. For this reason, there is likely to be a move in the future to fixed combination treatment, but certainly many patients with type 2 diabetes will require two, three or even four antihypertensives to get down to target, particularly where there is evidence of other complications, including renal disease.

It is also important to emphasise that the evidence base for cardiac and renal protection with ACE inhibitors and ARBs is at the higher doses of these agents, which should normally be used for maintenance after titration. ACE inhibitors and ARBs can also be used in combination as there is an additive affect on blood pressure lowering, although it is normally best to use combinations from different antihypertensive classes, reserving this particular combination for the most resistant cases.

KEY LEARNING POINTS
Approximately 80% of patients with diabetes are hypertensive based on the BHS guidelines (≥140/90mmHg)
The primary objective is to get the blood pressure down and to keep it down
When choosing an antihypertensive agent, all classes should be considered, although certain classes of antihypertensive may be preferred as first- or second-line
Most hypertensive patients will require multiple antihypertensive therapies to get down to target blood pressures

5 Diabetes, hyperglycaemia and cardiovascular disease

Even in the absence of other major cardiovascular risk factors, diabetes *per se* is associated with a significantly increased cardiovascular risk in both type 1 and type 2 diabetes. Hyperglycaemia *per se* adversely affects vascular endothelium and insulin resistance itself may be causally related. Until 1998, proof that improvement of diabetic control would be associated with reduction of vascular risk was circumstantial. This was, in part, through extrapolation of studies which showed that patients with poorer diabetic control have an increased risk of vascular, including cardiovascular, disease.

The United Kingdom Prospective Diabetes Study (UKPDS) randomised over 5,000 newly diagnosed type 2 diabetic patients into a conventionally treated and intensively treated group[7]. This study, lasting 20 years, was the largest and most intensive ever carried out in this area and achieved a separation of HbA_{1c} in favour of intensive treatment of 0.9%. This was associated with significant risk reductions for principally microvascular endpoints, including retinopathy and nephropathy (Table 4.2). There was also a reduction in risk for myocardial infarction, but this did not quite reach clinical significance. Epidemiological extrapolation of this data, however, suggests that for every 1% reduction in HbA_{1c} significant reductions in vascular events, including cardiovascular events, would be expected. This study allayed any doubts that improvement in glycaemic control would not be associated with long-term vascular benefit in patients with type 2 diabetes. It also supported an earlier study, the Diabetes Control and Complications Trial (DCCT), which again showed the profound benefits of intensified glycaemic control in type 1 diabetes from the point of view of microvascular benefit[86].

Management of hyperglycaemia

Diet and other lifestyle measures, including increased activity, still remain an important part of the holistic approach to the management of type 2 diabetes. However, the UKPDS showed that diet alone would be successful long term in under 10% of patients. This has led to the view that drug treatment for type 2 diabetes should not be long delayed, although pharmacotherapy should always be given in concert with lifestyle advice. Recommended glycaemic targets are generally based on HbA_{1c} and the overall message is to try and get HbA_{1c} down to < 7%.

Each drug class is considered in turn:

Biguanides

Metformin is the only drug of this class in use. Its exact mode of action is unknown, although it does inhibit hepatic glucose output and there is some evidence for a mild insulin sensitising effect[87]. The UKPDS showed cardiovascular benefit in obese type 2 diabetics treated with metformin compared with conventional therapy[88] (Fig 5.1). For this reason, metformin should be the usual first-line treatment in patients who are overweight (in practice the great majority), followed by fairly rapid progression to combination treatment where targets are still not being met. Its main side effects are gastrointestinal disturbance and it should therefore be started at low dosage with a gradual build-up to a reasonable maintenance dose of around 2g/day, divided as a twice-daily dosage. It should also be taken with or just after food. The extremely rare, but commonly fatal (if it does occur) side effect of lactic acidosis means that the drug is contraindicated in patients with significant renal, hepatic or cardiac impairment.

Sulphonylureas

These agents promote insulin secretion from the pancreatic beta-cells[87]. There are a whole range of such agents including glibenclamide, gliclazide, glipizide and tolbutamide. The major concerns with these agents are hypoglycaemia and weight gain and for these reasons the longer-acting agents such as glibenclamide should be avoided in elderly patients. These agents can be used for first-line treatment in patients who are of normal weight, but are usually used in combination with metformin in those not achieving HbA_{1c} targets.

Alpha-glucosidase inhibitors

These agents were introduced in the 1980s; the only one in use in the UK is acarbose. They act by inhibition of intestinal brush border enzymes thereby inhibiting the breakdown of long chain sugars to glucose in the gut[89]. They are not particularly efficacious in reducing HbA_{1c}, but do have significant effects on reduction in post-prandial hyperglycaemia. They have a high incidence of mainly gastrointestinal side effects, which can occur in over 50% of patients. Today, they

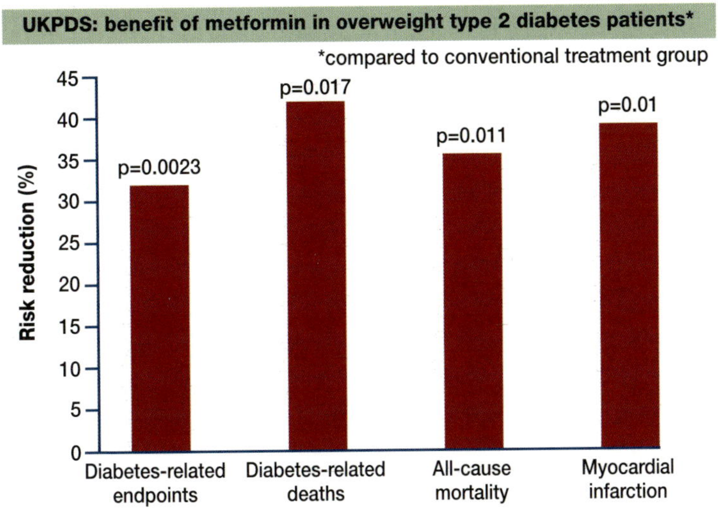

Fig 5.1 Demonstrates the cardiovascular benefits in obese type 2 diabetic patients treated with metformin compared with conventional therapy (adapted with from UKPDS 34. *Lancet* 1998[88] with permission from Elsevier).

are not commonly used in the UK and when they are, this is normally in combination treatment with other oral agents.

Rapid-acting insulin secretagogues

These agents include repaglinide and nateglinide. They act in a similar fashion to sulphonylureas in that they promote insulin secretion from the pancreas. They more specifically appear to target first-phase insulin secretion, which is lost very early in the disease process[90] (Fig 5.2). These agents, particularly nateglinide, restore first-phase insulin secretion, at least in part, thereby reducing post-prandial hyperglycaemia largely through inhibition of hepatic glucose output.

Repaglinide can be used as a monotherapy, but the normal use of these agents is in combination; indeed nateglinide is only licensed for use in combination with metformin. Given that metformin principally reduces fasting hyperglycaemia and nateglinide post-prandial hyperglycaemia, the combination can be quite powerful in reducing HbA_{1c}[91].

The use of agents that reduce post-prandial hyperglycaemia has gained some interest given that there is known to be an association between post-prandial hyperglycaemia and cardiovascular risk/mortality[92] (Fig 5.3). Whether this is causal is still debated and long-term trials are underway to try and answer the question as to whether reduction in post-prandial hyperglycaemia will reduce cardiovascular risk.

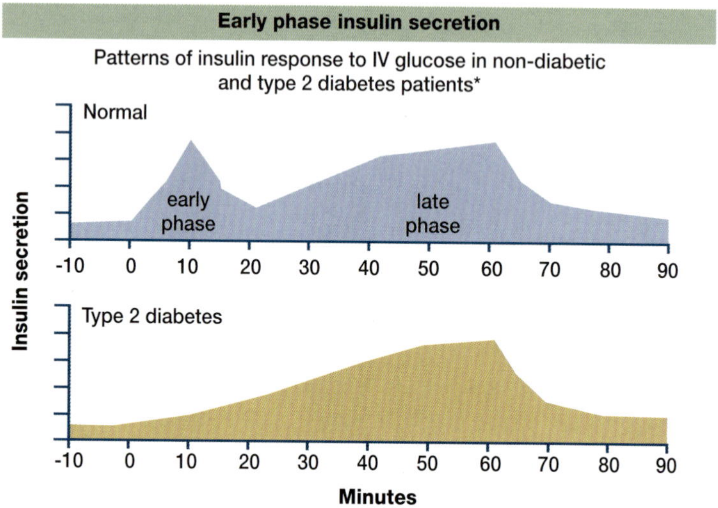

Fig 5.2 Demonstrates loss of early phase insulin secretion after an intravenous glucose load in type 2 diabetic patients compared with non-diabetic patients (adapted with permission from Davies M, 2002[90]).

A significant issue with these agents is that they need to be taken just before a meal (ie three times daily). This may increase compliance problems, although as these agents work by targeting post-prandial hyperglycaemia, their use in this way is logical – directly targeting the fundamental defect of type 2 diabetes. More physiological insulin profiles result with reduced risk of hypoglycaemia and less weight gain compared with standard sulphonylureas[93].

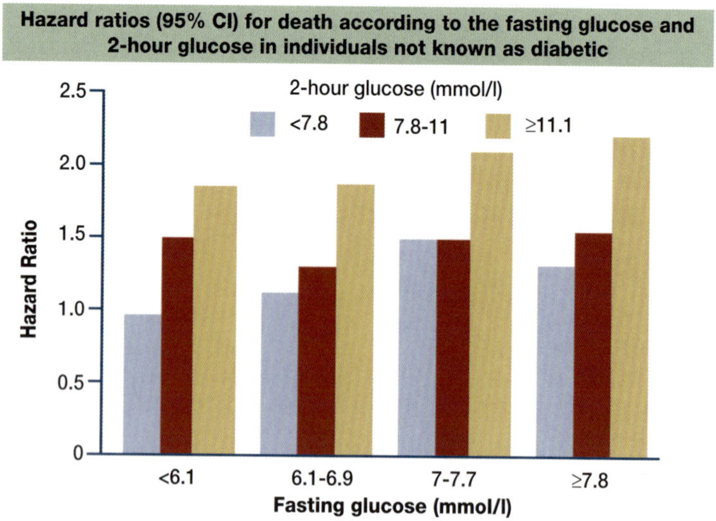

Fig 5.3 Demonstrates the relationship between post-prandial hyperglycaemia and mortality (mainly cardiovascular) in the DECODE study (adapted from DECODE Study Group. *Lancet* 1999[92] with permission from Elsevier).

These agents are useful where there are concerns about weight gain and hypoglycaemia, and may certainly be safer in 'missed meal' situations where giving a long-acting drug such as glibenclamide might provoke hypoglycaemia later in the day. As such they may be particularly useful for diabetic patients with erratic lifestyles where regular meals are not possible. In addition, nateglinide is glucose sensitive and if taken in the absence of food its effect is much attenuated, again reducing the risks of hypoglycaemia.

They may also be particularly useful early in the disease process and their role in disease prevention in patients with impaired glucose tolerance is presently being studied. The tantalising possibility of reduction of cardiovascular risk is also of great interest.

Thiazolidinediones (glitazones)

These agents have been on the market for a few years and are starting to make a significant impact. They act as insulin sensitisers thereby improving insulin sensitivity and reducing insulin resistance, a fundamental defect of type 2 diabetes[94]. For these reasons, they may also be useful agents in the management of the metabolic syndrome, although further research in this area is needed.

Thiazolidinediones work by combining with an intra-nuclear hormone receptor called peroxizome proliferator activated receptor gamma (PPARγ) (Fig 5.4). This interaction results in effects on carbohydrate and lipid metabolism, fat cell differentiation and gene regulation similar to that which occurs when insulin combines with its receptor[94]. Hence, these agents have an insulin sensitising effect, thereby reducing insulin resistance.

Early work in diabetic rodent models has demonstrated profound benefits both from the point of view of preservation of islet cells and improvement in glycaemia and lipids[95]. It was also noted that these agents did not cause hypoglycaemia and did not work in non-diabetic animals. Human studies have shown that these agents do improve insulin resistance both as monotherapy and in combination with metformin and sulphonylureas[96-99]. They have also been shown to improve pancreatic beta-cell function[96-99] and therefore appear to target both of the fundamental defects of type 2 diabetes.

In the human situation they have been shown to improve HbA_{1c} both as a monotherapy and in combination with traditional agents[94,97-99]. The present European licence allows glitazones to be used as a monotherapy where metformin is contraindicated or poorly tolerated. They are also particularly recommended in over-

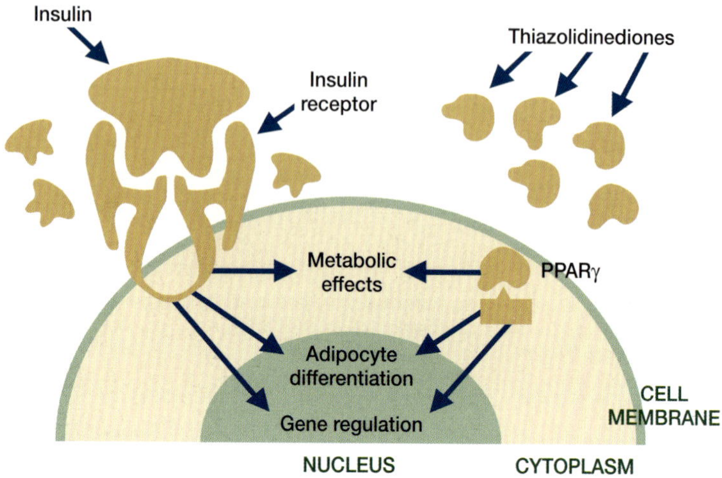

Fig 5.4 Demonstrates the mechanism of action of glitazones by combining with an intra-nuclear hormone receptor (PPARγ) resulting in effects on carbohydrate and lipid metabolism, fat cell differentiation and gene regulation similar to that which occurs when insulin combines with its receptor. These agents therefore have an insulin sensitising effect thereby reducing insulin resistance.

weight patients who are likely to be insulin resistant. Their major use in Europe remains in combination with either metformin or sulphonylurea in those who are not reaching target on a single agent. They are also used as triple therapy, although this is presently not a licensed combination.

The European licence states that insulin combination with the glitazones is a contraindication, although this is not the case in the

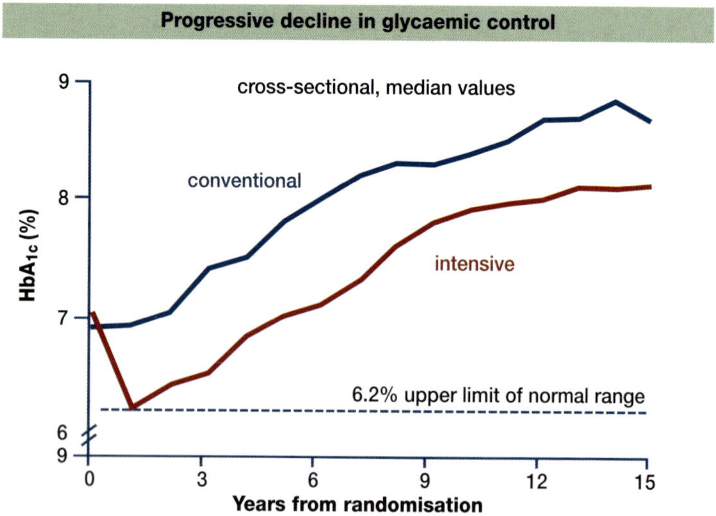

Fig 5.5 Demonstrates the fact that type 2 diabetes is a progressive disease as demonstrated by UKPDS and that none of the traditional agents which include sulphonylureas, metformin or insulin significantly affect that disease progression (adapted from UKPDS 33. *Lancet* 1998[7] with permission from Elsevier).

US and further studies are ongoing to try and extend the licence to this indication.

Why are new oral agents required?

Generally, the introduction of the glitazone class of drugs has been welcomed as a new approach to therapy for type 2 diabetes. This is in part because type 2 diabetes is a progressive disease and traditional agents such as metformin, sulphonylureas and insulin do not affect that progression[7] (Fig 5.5). In addition, all traditional agents have potential side effects: hypoglycaemia and weight gain with sulphonylureas and insulin; and gastrointestinal side effects with metformin. It has also become apparent from the UKPDS that the great majority of patients with type 2 diabetes will not manage long term on a single agent and will need combination therapy[7]. Thus, to have more drugs to choose from is to be welcomed. In addition, the ability to more directly target the two fundamental defects of type 2 diabetes (insulin secretory abnormalities and insulin resistance) is very attractive (Fig 5.6).

One might expect that an agent that improved insulin resistance would also improve other aspects of the metabolic syndrome; indeed there is evidence that the glitazones have a mild blood pressure reducing effect[100-101]. They also appear to have beneficial effects on the lipid profile. Pioglitazone, in particular, has been shown to reduce triglycerides with an increase in HDL cholesterol[94,97,98]

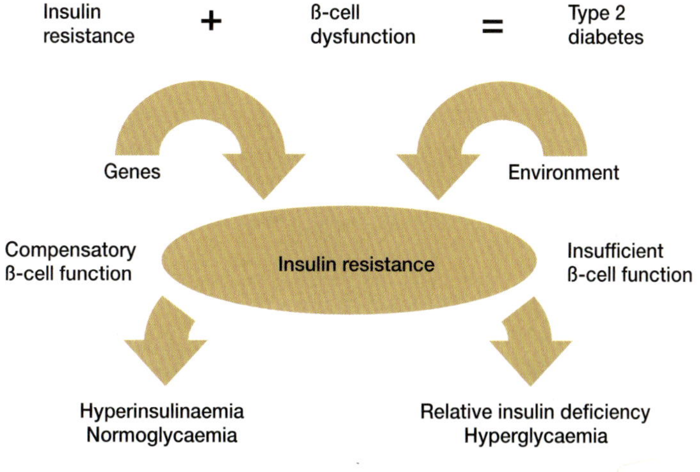

Fig 5.6 Demonstrates that both insulin secretory defects and insulin resistance are normally required for the development of type 2 diabetes.

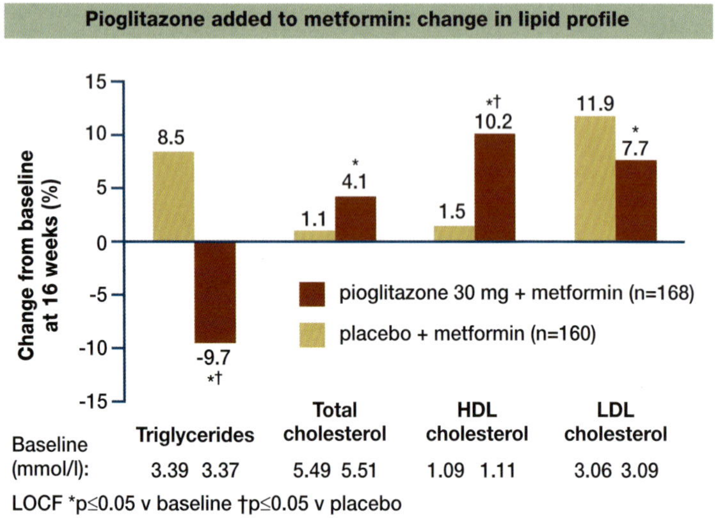

Fig 5.7a
Demonstrates the effects of the glitazone, pioglitazone, on the lipid profile in combination with metformin (adapted with permission from Einhorn D, et al. *Clin Ther* 2000[97]).

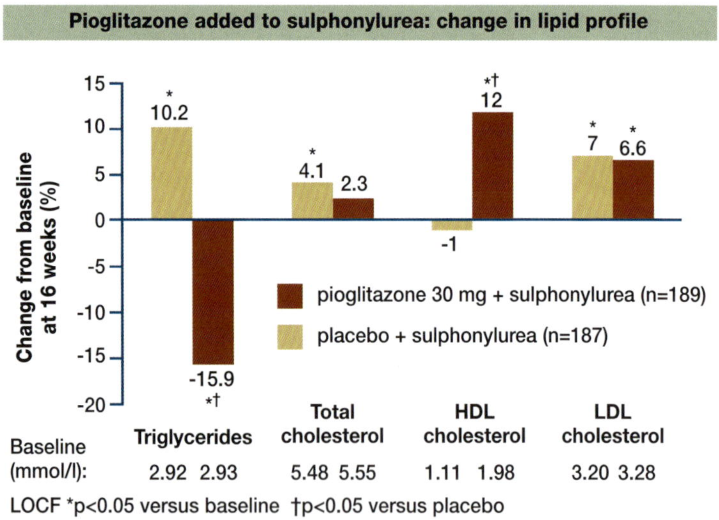

Fig 5.7b
Demonstrates the effects of the glitazone, pioglitazone, on the lipid profile in combination with sulphonylureas over a four month period. There is increase in HDL cholesterol and reduction in triglycerides (adapted with permission from Kipnes MS, et al. *Am J Med* 2001[98]).

(Fig 5.7a and 5.7b). The results for rosiglitazone are more controversial, although an increase in HDL cholesterol has been demonstrated[94]. There is also evidence for both glitazones of an increase in the light, less atherogenic lipoprotein particles and a reduction in small dense LDL atherogenic particles[94].

The glitazones have also more recently been shown to improve surrogate markers of cardiovascular risk, which include markers of

Fig 5.8 Demonstrates reduction in carotid intima-media thickness with pioglitazone (adapted from Koshiyama HM, et al. *J Clin Endocrinol Metab* 2001; 86(7): 3452-56).

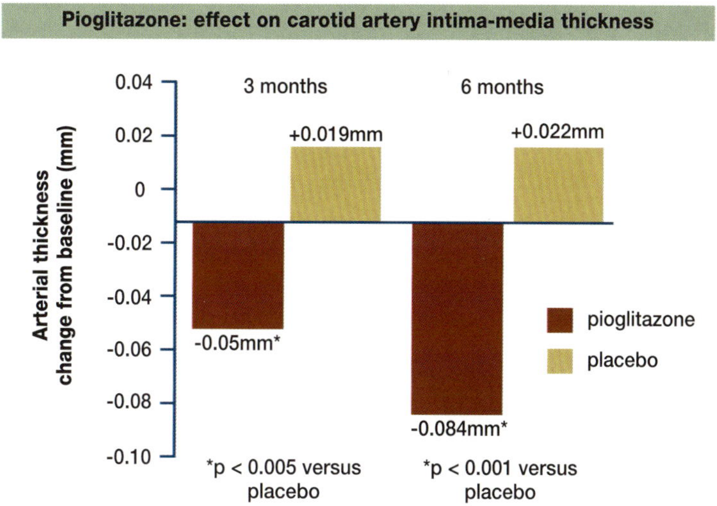

endothelial cell dysfunction such as microalbuminuria, inflammation (CRP) and clotting (PAI-1)[94]. A significant reduction in carotid artery intima-media thickness in diabetic patients has also been demonstrated (Fig 5.8).

Several studies are presently ongoing to answer two fundamental questions:

- Will the glitazones prevent type 2 diabetes and also reduce disease progression when it becomes established? There is a sound theoretical basis to suggest this and the results are awaited with interest.
- Through their effects on insulin resistance will these agents reduce cardiovascular risk? Again, this question is the subject of large scale, hard endpoint trials.

Safety

The glitazones initially were given a bad press due to the finding of idiosyncratic hepatotoxicity leading to liver failure and death in around 1-in-50,000 patients on troglitazone, the originally marketed agent[94]. It appears, however, that this is a property only seen with troglitazone and is possibly related to its overall structure which includes a vitamin E moiety that 'homes in' on the liver. The quinone metabolite of troglitazone is thought to be the reason for the idiosyncratic reactions. Neither rosiglitazone nor

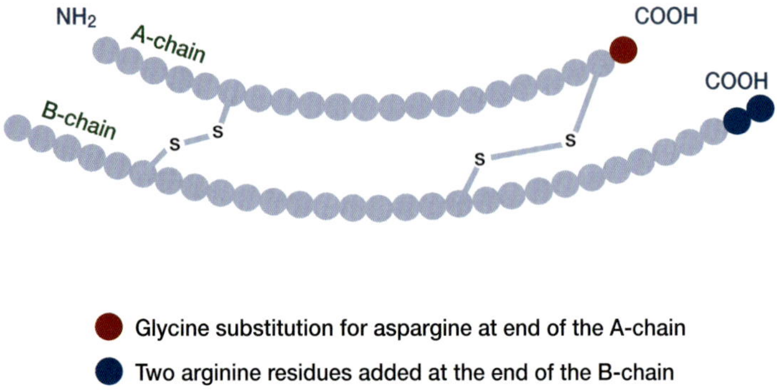

Fig 5.9 Demonstrates the structure of the new long-acting insulin analogues, insulin glargine.

pioglitazone possess the vitamin E moiety and usage over long periods in many millions of patients now testifies to the safety of these agents, with no evidence for hepatic toxicity.

Other concerns include weight gain, which as a class effect is around 3-5kg in the first six months of treatment, which then stabilises[94]. This is in part due to a re-distribution from intra-abdominal fat stores to peripheral fat stores; something which may be of advantage in the context of the metabolic syndrome. Indeed, any weight gain appears not to be associated with a deterioration in cardiovascular risk markers: there is, in fact, an improvement.

There is also a 5% incidence of peripheral oedema[94]. Although this is not usually a significant problem, it occasionally necessitates discontinuation of the drug. Because of the potential for fluid retention, these drugs are contraindicated in patients with a history of heart failure, although again the European licence differs from the US licence where the latter only cites contraindication in the more severe forms of heart failure. There is a suggestion that the combination of glitazone with insulin is associated with more fluid retention and this is one of the reasons why this combination is contraindicated in Europe. Despite using the same data, the US has not interpreted this in the same way. Indeed, the combination of glitazones with insulin has been shown to be very powerful in reducing insulin requirements and improving HbA_{1c}[102].

A further offshoot of this technology is the study of other agents that may act in a similar way. There are now several studies looking at agonists of both PPARγ and PPARα. These agents would be expected to show similar benefits to glitazones, but with more profound effects on the lipid profile.

Insulin

Given that type 2 diabetes is a progressive disease with an increasing requirement for improvement in glycaemic control, insulin therapy is now commonly used in the management of type 2 diabetes. For patients failing on combination oral treatment, there is now a vogue for adding a single long-acting basal insulin injection[99]. With the advent of the new long-acting insulin analogues, which include insulin glargine (Fig 5.9) and insulin detemir, this becomes a particularly useful possibility. Insulin glargine has a 24-hour profile and is associated with a reduced risk of nocturnal hypoglycaemia and perhaps less weight gain compared with traditional basal insulins. Insulin detemir may also have similar clinical advantages, but is not yet on the market. Insulin glargine can be given either in the morning or at bedtime as a supplement to oral agents (metformin and sulphonylurea), which are continued. This has been associated with improvements in HbA_{1c} and patient well-being[103].

Where there is still insufficient glycaemic control then the alternative is to proceed to twice daily pre-mixed insulin of rapid-acting and basal insulin, often used in combination with metformin, or alternatively a basal bolus regimen involving pre-prandial rapid-acting insulin together with a basal insulin either at bedtime or in the morning, again commonly in association with metformin.

One thing is certain, many patients have been denied the benefits of insulin therapy due to the mistaken belief that the health professional is in some way preserving the quality of life of the

Fig 5.10 Percentage HbA_{1c} comparing 3-month treatment between subcutaneous and inhaled insulin in patients with type 1 diabetes showing fall in HbA_{1c} but no significant difference between the groups (reproduced from Skyler JS et al. *Lancet* 2001[106] with permission from Elsevier).

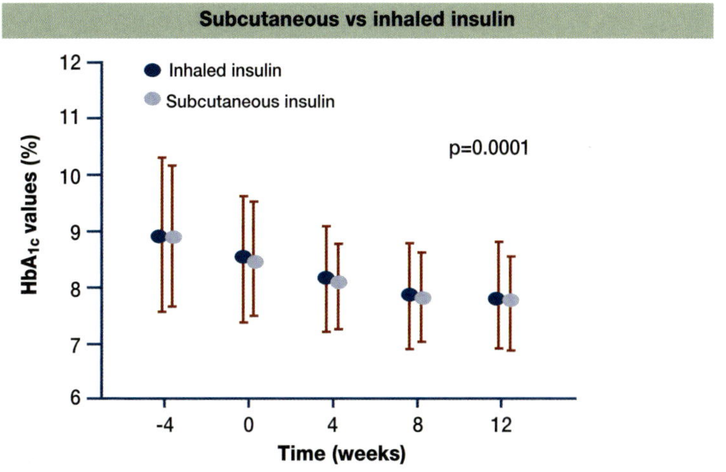

patient. In practice, many patients have suffered years of symptoms and ill-health through this attitude.

Alternative insulin delivery systems

There is presently much interest in inhaled insulin. The large surface area and high permeability of the lung suggests this as an ideal delivery route for insulin[104]. The first inhaled insulin to come to market is likely to be the product developed by Inhaled Therapeutic Systems for which Pfizer and Aventis are currently conducting phase III clinical trials. Inhaled insulin has a more rapid onset of action than subcutaneously injected insulin and appears at least as good as standard soluble insulins from the point of view of glycaemic control[105-106] (Fig 5.10). It also has high patient acceptability. In one study of patients with type 2 diabetes, inadequately controlled on oral hypoglycaemics, the addition of inhaled insulin pre-prandially was associated with significantly greater reductions in HbA_{1c} than oral therapy alone[107].

The studies have shown no increased incidence of hypoglycaemia, but there is concern whether the long-term inhalation of insulin might have deleterious effects on the lung. Evidence is still limited, but is not suggestive of a significant problem. Indeed, inhaled insulin might improve patient compliance and encourage more people with type 2 diabetes to start treatment, which is often necessary. Presently, the only inhaled insulins in significant development are rapid-acting formulations. Long-acting formulations also need to be considered if we are to totally abolish the need for subcutaneous injections.

KEY LEARNING POINTS
Improving control of glycaemia is vital for the prevention of long-term vascular complications and improved quality of life in patients with type 2 diabetes
Metformin is recommended first-line for overweight/obese diabetic patients. Sulphonylureas are used first-line in patients who are of normal weight and in combination with metformin in patients not achieving HbA_{1c} targets (<7%)
Newer agents are now available that directly target the fundamental defects of type 2 diabetes – insulin resistance and beta-cell dysfunction
Insulin therapy is commonly used in the management of type 2 diabetes and can be used in combination with oral therapy
New delivery methods are being developed for insulin. These may improve patient compliance and encourage more patients to start treatment

6 Diabetes and non-classical cardiovascular risk factors

Although diabetes, hypertension, dyslipidaemia, cigarette smoking, family history and central obesity appear to be the major risk factors for cardiovascular disease, there has been much recent interest in the so called non-classical risk factors. Diabetes itself is a prothrombotic state associated with increased blood viscosity, defects in coagulation and fibrinolysis and reduced blood flow in the microcirculatory system[108].

Other risk markers include raised fibrinogen and increased plasminogen activator inhibitor 1 (PAI-1) activity. The finding of microalbuminuria (an albumin excretion rate above the normal range but below the level of dipstick detection) is not only a marker of 'leaky' kidneys, but also signifies a generalised endothelial pathology and is itself associated with greatly increased cardiovascular risk[6]. Markers of inflammation such as C-reactive protein (CRP) have also been shown to be increased in the context of diabetes and cardiovascular risk.

It is of interest that the recently marketed glitazones appear to show beneficial effects on these parameters, perhaps through insulin sensitisation, although the exact mechanism is still unclear. Hard endpoint trials are presently being conducted to determine if this will be reflected in cardiovascular benefit.

KEY LEARNING POINTS

- Diabetes is a prothrombotic state associated with changes in coagulation
- Microalbuminuria has been shown to be a risk factor for cardiovascular disease in people with diabetes
- A number of other risk markers have been identified including raised fibrinogen, increased PA1-1 activity, and increased markers of inflammation (CRP)
- Glitazones appear to show beneficial effects on these non-classical risk factors, although further research in this area is needed

7 Organising diabetes care in general practice

New GP contract

The organisation of good quality care for people with diabetes is a medical, financial and administrative challenge, but is now an epidemiological imperative. The new GMS (General Medical Services) GP contract (GMS2) prioritises the care of people with diabetes, hypertension and coronary heart disease by 'rewarding' the practice with a relatively high number of payment-linked quality points[109]. These are intended to reflect the degree to which the practice team carries out a regular review of these patients and provides evidence-based care. With support from primary care trusts (PCTs), primary and secondary care teams are being motivated to work together to develop locally sensitive services for their diabetic populations. Although the new GP contract helps to concentrate the minds of those planning and providing care, and appears to go some way towards proper remuneration for the work done, the exploding prevalence rates and relative manpower shortage will continue to be a considerable challenge.

Improving standards of diabetes care

Over the past 20 years there has been a wealth of articles published in the UK and worldwide documenting the successes and failures of the many schemes set up to deliver diabetes care. Diabetes care has moved from large, impersonal hospital-based diabetes clinics to a 'shared care' model with increasing involvement of primary care services. The success of various schemes depends not just on the availability of clinical expertise, but also on the organisational and administrative support that underpins the diabetes service.

The Audit Commission review of diabetes services in England and Wales[110] provides evidence for the broad state of services in 2000. It applauds the many excellent examples of collaborative and innovative care, but also highlights the deficiencies and failures of some services (Table 7.1). The National Service Framework documents for diabetes[13,111] have responded to these findings and provide guidance on the key elements of good diabetes care. The original NSF for Diabetes published 12 standards, which included standards on the prevention of type 2 diabetes; screening for diabetes;

empowerment of people with diabetes; care of adults; care of children and the young; diabetic emergencies; inpatient diabetes management; pregnancy; and long-term complications. These standards were followed by a delivery strategy document in 2002 with a commencement date in 2003[13]. The NSF is a 10-year programme and at the end of this time, it is expected that all the standards will be met.

In addition, certain priorities have been set: for example, 80% of people with diabetes should have systematic retinopathy screening and necessary treatment by 2006. By 2007 this will be 100%. In primary care, by March 2006, there must be in place practice-based registers and systematic treatment regimens including appropriate advice on diet, physical activity and smoking. This should also cover most patients at risk of cardiovascular disease, particularly those with hypertension, diabetes and those with a BMI >30. The disease register databases should be linked to education and treatment protocols.

Table 7.1 Key messages from the Audit Commission review, Testing Times

- The number of people with diabetes in the UK is expected to increase from 1.4 million to 3 million by the year 2010 and there is an absence of strategic planning for this rise in service demand
- Diabetes is 3 to 4 times more common in people of Asian and Afro-Caribbean origin
- Up to half of people with diabetes are thought to be undiagnosed
- The incidence of type 2 diabetes can be reduced by preventative health strategies
- Diabetes consumes a very large slice of the country's health budget – hospital costs for a person with diabetes are six times higher than for a person without diabetes
- Services are already stretched, but duplication and lack of organisation of care is aggravating this
- Little cost-effectiveness research has been done, although there is clear evidence on what works in diabetes care. Good care prevents or reduces complications

Hospital Services

- The majority of hospitals could not produce information on how many patients had received a recent full review
- Few hospitals had dedicated psychological support for people with diabetes
- Less than half the hospitals visited had comprehensive programmes of patient education
- The services for ethnic minority groups were inadequate
- Patients frequently reported the feeling that the consultation was too rushed

Primary Care

- Most patients are being managed in primary care but standards vary hugely
- Over one-third of practices had no referral guidelines for their patients with diabetes
- Nurses alone run one-third of diabetic clinics
- Less than one-third of practices had access to a dietitian or podiatrist

The 'empowerment' of patients with diabetes will enable them to make informed decisions about their care and be proactive in participating in education programmes. This will facilitate more self-care and is essential if we are to manage the explosion in diabetes and cardiovascular disease across the globe. It also means that the experience of illness will be less alienating for patients and they will have an improved quality of life.

The new GP contract recognises that diabetes care is a major commitment for the general practice team. It attracts 99 points in the quality league, outscored only by cardiovascular disease and hypertension. It has the greatest number of indicators of any clinical domain (in total 18) and meeting these will thoroughly test even the most organised practice (Table 7.2). Primary care teams will need to know exactly where and how all the required elements of diabetes care are being provided for their patients. They must be able to easily access and track clinical and biochemical information, ensuring transmission to the PCT and thus payment of their salaries. However, this is not just about reinventing the wheel: the organised application of well-known principles of diabetes care will produce 'the points' and, in turn, a much healthier diabetes population.

The multidisciplinary team: evolving and expanding

One of the problems that has beset diabetes care in the past has been the polarisation of primary and secondary care. This professional 'territorialism' meant that the seamless care, which was the ideal of many, rarely happened. It is all too easy to stereotype the specialists and the generalists, failing to recognise the essential strengths of each. The person with diabetes needs the skills of both groups. Strategic discussions that include expressions like 'shifting care' are implicitly negative and demoralising for people 'working on the ground' in primary and secondary care.

The provision of good diabetes care is complex. There are few other diseases where patients have to negotiate such a complicated care pathway. With the development of macrovascular and microvascular complications, the life of some diabetic patients is punctuated by frequent visits to their GP practice as well as frequent hospital appointments to see a myriad of professionals. It is easy to understand how people can get 'lost to care' and demotivated if they do not form supportive and meaningful relationships with these professionals. Patients need to feel confident that there is a reliable communication system between all those involved in their

Table 7.2: Indicators for diabetes (GMS2)

Diabetes Mellitus (Diabetes)

This set of indicators refers to patients with both type 1 and type 2 diabetes.

Indicator	Points	Payment stages
Records		
DM 1.The practice can produce a register of all patients with diabetes mellitus	6	
Ongoing Management		
DM 2.The percentage of patients with diabetes whose notes record BMI in the previous 15 months	3	25-90%
DM 3. The percentage of patients with diabetes in whom there is a record of smoking status in the previous 15 months, except those who have never smoked where smoking status should be recorded once	3	25-90%
DM 4. The percentage of patients with diabetes who smoke and whose notes contain a record that smoking cessation advice or referral to a specialist service, where available, has been offered in the last 15 months	5	25-90%
DM 5. The percentage of diabetic patients who have a record of HbA_{1C} or equivalent in the previous 15 months	3	25-90%
DM 6. The percentage of patients with diabetes in whom the last HbA_{1C} is 7.4 or less (or equivalent test/reference range depending on local laboratory) in last 15 months	16	25-50%
DM 7. The percentage of patients with diabetes in whom the last HbA_{1C} is 10 or less (or equivalent test/reference range depending on local laboratory) in last 15 months	11	25-85%
DM 8. The percentage of patients with diabetes who have a record of retinal screening in the previous 15 months	5	25-90%
DM 9.The percentage of patients with diabetes with a record of the presence or absence of peripheral pulses in the previous 15 months	3	25-90%
DM 10. The percentage of patients with diabetes with a record of neuropathy testing in the previous 15 months	3	25-90%

care – a reality if integrated care is accessible, efficient and empowering. The multidisciplinary team (see Table 7.3) should straddle primary and secondary care and be free from the organisational constraints and financial arrangements that have, in the past, smothered good clinical practice and lead to duplication. The diabetes specialist nurse, podiatrist, link-worker and dietitian should be accessible to the patient regardless of whether or not they are registered with a hospital clinic. PCTs now have their own diabetes 'departments' where community diabetes services are organised and communication between hospital departments is improving at an accelerated rate. Service and educational support resources are now moving in a two-way direction. In addition, clinical skills in diabetes are improving due to the many diabetes accreditation courses now provided across the UK. Diabetes teams are becoming more creative in their approach to patient education and empowerment and lifestyle issues are being tackled in a less medicalised way using more locally relevant programmes: an area that is seen as one of the most challenging aspects of the problems of diabetes care.

Community diabetologists are now being appointed by many PCTs and are key figures in developing services that are appropriate

Table 7.3: The multidisciplinary team

- Diabetes specialist nurse
- Dietitian
- Podiatrist
- Practice nurse
- Primary care physician
- Hospital-based diabetologist
- District nurse
- Optometrist
- Link worker
- Community-based diabetologist
- Community-based nurse consultant

Table 7.4: Role of the community diabetologist

- Assess the size of the diabetes population in the district
- Introduce and maintain a district diabetes register
- Work with the PCT to plan a locally relevant, patient-centred service
- Offer accessible clinical support to primary care physicians
- Liaise with local hospital services to encourage their needs-based development
- Organise educational programmes that will foster a spirit of collaboration across primary and secondary care
- Encourage community-based research
- Act as an advocate for adequate resources especially for primary care

to local needs. Ideally such people should have experience of working in both primary and secondary care and act as a senior and key bridge between the two disciplines. Table 7.4 illustrates their key roles.

Providing a diabetes service

The new GP contract outlines the following standards of care for patients with diabetes.

Diabetes register

All general practices will need to maintain an up-to-date diabetes register. This will form the template for calculating all the other diabetic quality indicators. Patients under 16 are excluded as their follow-up is usually under hospital care; however, it should be noted that patients who reach the age of 16 by 1 April, the annual cut-off date for quality assessment, need to be registered. Patients with gestational diabetes and impaired glucose tolerance should not be included, although they will need to be kept under annual surveillance as some will go on to develop diabetes. Practice registers will allow easy compilation of district registers, which can then provide local population information on ethnicity, age profile, social class, demographic trends and ultimately prevalence rates for diabetes. This ensures 'needs-based' resource planning, especially important

Table 7.5: The diabetes annual review

Overall assessment of diabetes control	
Cardiovascular risk assessment calculation	
	Lipids (total cholesterol, HDL cholesterol, triglycerides)
	Blood pressure
	Smoking history/advice
Screening for complications	
Eyes	Visual acuity
	Pupillary dilatation
	Ophthalmoscopy
	Retinal photography (preferred method)
Kidneys	Proteinuria
	Microalbuminuria
	Blood pressure
Feet	Neuropathy
	Peripheral vascular disease

in those areas of the country where diabetes prevalence rates are double that of the national average of 2-4%.

Annual review

All people with diabetes require an annual review (Table 7.5) in order to pick up complications early. Eleven of the 18 diabetic quality indicators involve carrying out and recording some routine quality checks. These quality indicators are 'evidence based' and the rationale for the indicators is explained on pages 32-43 of 'Supporting Documentation for the New GMS Contract'[109]. The annual review can be carried out in a GP or hospital clinic and should be performed in a structured way, at a pace that allows time for patient education. Results of any investigations should be available, preferably through computerised hospital-GP surgery links. Some elements of the annual review require specialist services such as retinopathy screening and the results of these investigations should be integrated into a central recall system.

Dietetic and educational review

In general practice many of the tasks are delegated to practice nurses. Staff should be adequately trained in diabetes and have the necessary computing skills to input the data. Group practices will usually have a 'diabetes lead' doctor, who is responsible for overseeing the diabetes care in the practice. Practice managers have a key role in ensuring the smooth running of the planning, administration and resourcing of the diabetes service. Personalising care by making named receptionists responsible for organising appointments and chasing up diabetic defaulters can be helpful in improving patient compliance.

However successful a practice is in getting its diabetes patients to attend for their checks, the greater challenge lies in delivering optimal clinical outcomes. The quality framework offers 56 points for achieving the six outcome indicators. Extra appointments are generated for both the GP and practice nurse to monitor blood pressure, diabetes control, for example. The implications for overall workload are obvious. For practices with high prevalence rates for diabetes, efficiency will be the key to optimising income and resources for their diabetic population.

Patient empowerment

The approach to diabetes care in each practice should be patient-centred allowing the development of a service that suits the needs of the population. This approach is more likely to be successful in terms of compliance with appointments, treatment and lifestyle advice. Patients should be provided with clear, personalised written guidance on what their individual 'targets' are and what is expected of them. Group education sessions are a good way of facilitating fairly open patient discussion; this can also help patients to develop confidence and 'ownership' for their condition. The internet is now accessible to an increasing number of people in their homes and patients should be given addresses of websites where they can access information on diabetes, such as Diabetes UK (www.diabetes.org.uk).

Integrated care

The system of care depends on clinical need; specialist care should be integrated as specific groups of people will need hospital-based care[112]. These include children and adolescents with type 1 diabetes, pregnant women and those with established microvascular complications. Patients with type 2 diabetes who have microvascular complications and those on insulin will often need secondary and tertiary care at various stages in their disease. Where possible, reviews at specialist clinics (eg diabetes renal clinic, diabetes eye clinic) should be integrated with day-to-day diabetes care so that hospital appointments are more easily negotiated.

Audit and performance measurement

The quality targets in the new contract include all three principles of clinical audit: structure, process and outcome:

- **Structure** (six points) involves having an accurate patient register – a requirement common to all 10 chronic conditions.
- **Process** (32 points) involves completing clinical management tasks and most of these can be covered at the annual review.
- **Outcome** (56 points) involves demonstrating good standards of diabetes care – more difficult to achieve but best rewarded.

Conclusion

The new GP contract gives diabetes care prominence in the work of a primary care team. To achieve the best outcomes for patients with diabetes, a spirit of joint ownership of services must exist between the generalists and specialists involved in diabetes care. In most areas the skills and motivation are there to provide an excellent service, but these need to be organised appropriately. It is important that resources are considerably increased to maintain the ambitious standards set out in the new GP contract.

KEY LEARNING POINTS
The new GP contract prioritises the care of people with diabetes, hypertension and coronary heart disease
General practices are required to set up diabetes practice registers and provide an annual review of all patients with diabetes
Diabetes care should adopt an integrated care approach with a high degree of coordination between those working in primary and secondary care
Adequate resources are needed to meet the challenge of delivering effective care against a backdrop of increasing prevalence rates and manpower shortage

References

1. Zimmet PZ, McCarty DJ, de Courten MP. The global epidemiology of non-insulin-dependent diabetes mellitus and the metabolic syndrome. *J Diabetes Complications* 1997;11:60-68.
2. Barnett AH, Spiliopoulos AJ, Pyke DA et al. Muscle capillary basement membrane thickness in identical twins discordant for insulin-dependent diabetes. *Diabetes* 1983;32:557-60.
3. British Diabetic Association, Diabetes in the UK – 1996. London: British Diabetic Association, 1995.
4. World Health Organization (Europe) and International Diabetes Federation (Europe). Diabetes care and research in Europe: the St Vincent declaration. *Diabet Med* 1990;7:360-70.
5. Currie CJ, Kraus D, Morgan CL et al. NHS acute sector expenditure for diabetes: the present, future and excess in-patient cost of care. *Diabet Med* 1997;14:686-92.
6. O'Donnell MJ, Chowdhury TA. Hypertension and nephropathy in diabetes. In: Barnett AH, Dodson PM. *Hypertension and Diabetes* (3rd Edn). London: Science Press Ltd 2000; 21-31.
7. United Kingdom Prospective Diabetes Study (UKPDS) Group. Intensive blood glucose control with sulphonylureas or insulin compared with conventional treatment and risk of complications in patients with type 2 diabetes (UKPDS 33). *Lancet* 1998;352:837-53.
8. United Kingdom Prospective Diabetes Study Group. Tight blood pressure control and risk of macrovascular and microvascular complications in type 2 diabetes: UKPDS 38. *BMJ* 1998:317:703-13.
9. Hansson L, Zanchetti A, Carruthers SG et al. Effect of intensive blood pressure lowering and low-dose aspirin in patients with hypertension: principal results of the Hypertension Optimal Treatment (HOT) randomised trial. *Lancet* 1998;351:1755-62.
10. Pyorala K, Pedersen TR, Kjekshus J et al. Cholesterol lowering with simvastatin improves prognosis of diabetic patients with coronary heart disease. *Diabetes Care* 1997;20:614-20.
11. Heart Protection Study Collaborative Group. MRC/BHF Heart Protection study of cholesterol lowering with simvastatin in 20,536 high risk individuals: a randomised placebo-controlled trial. *Lancet* 2002;360:7-22.
12. National Institute for Clinical Excellence. Management of type 2 diabetes – management of blood pressure and blood lipids. Integrated Clinical Guideline H. London, Oct 2002.
13. National Service Framework (NSF) for Diabetes : Delivery Strategy. London; Department of Health 2003.
14. National Service Framework for Coronary Heart Disease. London: Department of Health, 2000.
15. Ramsay L, Williams B, Johnston G et al. Guidelines for management of hypertension: report of the third working party of the British Hypertension Society. *J Human Hypertens* 1999;13:569-92.
16. Kannel WB and McGee DL. Diabetes and cardiovascular risk factors: the Framingham study. *Circulation* 1979;59(1):8-13.
17. Fisher M, Shaw KM. Diabetes – a state of premature cardiovascular death. *Pract Diab Int* 2001;18:183-84.
18. Stamler J, Vaccaro O, Neaton JD, Wentworth D. Diabetes, other risk factors and 12-year mortality for men as screened in the multiple risk factor intervention trial. *Diabetes Care* 1993;16(2):434-44.
19. Tzagournis M. Interaction of diabetes with hypertension and lipids – patients at high risk. An overview. *Am J Med* 1989;86:50-54.
20. Dodson PM, Barnett AH. *Lipids, Diabetes and Vascular Disease* (2nd Edn) London: Science Press, 1998.
21. Haffner SM, Lehto S, Ronnemaa T et al. Mortality from coronary heart disease in subjects with type 2 diabetes and in non-diabetic subjects with and without prior myocardial infarction. *New Eng J Med* 1998;339:229-34.
22. Pan WH, Cedres LB, Liu K et al. Relationship of clinical diabetes and asymptomatic hyperglycemia to risk of coronary heart disease mortality in men and women. *Am J Epidemiol* 1986;123:504-16.
23. Singer DE, Moulton AW, Nathan DM. Diabetic myocardial infarction. Interaction of diabetes with other preinfarction risk factors. *Diabetes* 1989;38:350-57.
24. American Diabetes Association. Direct and indirect costs of diabetes in the USA in 1992. Alexandria, VA: American Diaebtes Association,1993.
25. Songer T. The economic costs of NIDDM. *Diab Metab Rev* 1992;8:389-404.

26. Reaven GM. Role of insulin resistance in human disease: Banting Lecture. *Diabetes* 1988;37:1595-1607
27. British Nutrition Foundation. Obesity. Report of the British Nutrition Foundation Taskforce. Oxford: Blackwell Scientific Ltd 1999
28. Ford ES, Giles WH, Dietz WH. Prevalence of the metabolic syndrome among US adults: findings from the third National Health and Nutrition Examination Survey. *JAMA* 2002;287:356-59.
29. NCEP Expert Panel. Third report of the NCEP Expert Panel on Detection, Evaluation and Treatment of High Blood Cholesterol in Adults (ATPIII). Bethesda MD: National Institute of Health, 2002.
30. World Health Organization. Definition, diagnosis and classification of diabetes mellitus and its complications. Part 1. Diagnosis and classification of diabetes mellitus. Geneva: WHO: 1999.
31. Lapidus L, Bengtsson C, Larsson B et al. Distribution of adipose tissue and risk of cardiovascular disease and death: a 12 year follow up of participants in the population study of women in Gothenburg, Sweden. *BMJ* (Clin Res Ed) 1984;289:1257-61.
32. Larsson B, Svardsudd K, Welin L et al. Abdominal adipose tissue distribution, obesity, and risk of cardiovascular disease and death: 13 year follow up of participants in the study of men born in 1913. *BMJ* (Clin Res Ed) 1984;288:1401-04.
33. Office for Population Consensuses and Surveys. Health Survey for England. London; HMSO 1991.
34. Kuczmarski RJ, Flegal KM, Campbell SM, Johnson CL. Increasing prevalence of overweight among US adults. The National Health and Nutrition Examination Surveys 1960 to 1991. *JAMA* 1994; 272:205-11.
35. Calle EE, Thun MJ, Petrelli JM et al. Body mass index and mortality in a prospective cohort of U.S. adults. *New Engl J Med* 1999;341:1097-105.
36. World Health Organization. The Asia-Pacific perspective: redefining obesity and its treatment. Geneva: WHO 2000.
37. Wilding J, Williams G. Diabetes and obesity. In: Kopelman PG (ed). *Clinical Obesity*. Oxford: Blackwell Science 1998:308-49.
38. Group DPPR. Reduction in the incidence of type 2 diabetes with lifestyle intervention or metformin. *N Eng J Med* 2002;346:393-403.
39. Tuomilehto J, Lindstrom J, Eriksson J G et al. Prevention of type 2 diabetes mellitus by lifestyle among subjects with impaired glucose tolerance. *N Eng J Med* 2001;344:1343-50.
40. Torgerson JS, Hauptman J, Boldrin MN, Sjostrom L. XENical in the prevention of diabetes in obese subjects (XENDOS) study: a randomised study of orlistat as an adjunct to lifestyle changes for the prevention of type 2 diabetes in obese patients. *Diabetes Care* 2004;27(1):155-61.
41. Lean ME, Powrie JK, Anderson AS, Garthwaite PH. Obesity, weight loss and prognosis in type 2 diabetes. *Diabet Med* 1990;7:228-33.
42. Hanif MW, Kumar S. Pharmacological management of obesity. *Expert Opin Pharmacother* 2002;3:1711-18.
43. Allahabadia A, Kumar S. Diabetes and obesity: what is the relationship to cardiovascular disease? In: Barnett AH (ed). *Diabetes Annual.* London: Martin Dunitz 2002;15-39.
44. Scandinavian Simvastatin Survival Study Group. Randomised controlled trial of cholesterol lowering in 4444 patients with coronary heart disease: The Scandinavian Simvastatin Survival Study (4S). *Lancet* 1994;344:1383-89.
45. Shepherd J, Cobbs SM, Ford I et al. Prevention of coronary heart disease with pravastatin in men with hypercholesterolaemia. *N Engl J Med* 1995;333: 1301-07.
46. Sacks FM, Pfeffer MA, Moye LA et al. The effect of pravastatin on coronary events after myocardial infarction in patients with average cholesterol levels. *N Engl J Med* 1996;335:1001-09.
47. Downs JR, Clearfield M, Weis S et al. Primary prevention of acute coronary events with lovastatin in men and women with average cholesterol levels. Results of AFCAPS/TexCAPS. *JAMA* 1998;279: 1615-22.
48. The Long-Term Intervention with Pravastatin in Ischemic Disease (LIPID) Study Group. Prevention of cardiovascular events and death with pravastatin in patients with coronary heart disease and a broad range of initial cholesterol levels. *N Engl J Med* 1998;339:1349-57.
49. Colhoun HM, Thomason MJ, Mackness MI et al. Design of the Collaborative Atorvastatin Diabetes Study (CARDS) in patients with type 2 diabetes. *Diabetic Med* 2002; 19:201-11.
50. Athyros VG, Mikhailidis DP, Papageorgious AA, Mercouris BR et al. Attaining United Kingdom-European Atherosclerosis Society low density lipoprotein cholesterol guideline target values in the Greek Atorvastatin and Coronary-heart-disease Evaluation (GREACE) Study. *Curr Med Res Opin* 2002; 18(8): 499-502.
51. Athyros VG, Papageorgiou AA, Symeonidis AN et al; GREACE Study Collaborative Group. Early benefit from structured cae with atorvastatin in patients with coronary heart disease and diabetes mellitus. *Angiology* 2003; 54(6): 679-90.

52. Sever PS, Dehlof B, Poulter NR et al. Prevention of coronary and stroke events with atorvastatin in hypertensive patients who have average or lower than average cholesterol concentrations in the Anglo-Scandinavian Cardiac Outcomes Trial - Lipid Lowering Arm (ASCOT-LLA): a multicentre randomised controlled trial. *Lancet* 2003; 561:1149-56.
53. Minhas R. Current progress in lipid therapy. *Br J Cardiol* 2003;10:59-68.
54. Blasetto JW, Stein EA, Brown WV et al. Efficacy of rosuvastatin compared with other statins at selected starting doses in hypercholesterolemic patients and in special population groups. *Am J Cardiol* 2003; 91(suupl):3C-10C.
55. Olsson AG, Pears J, McKellar et al. Effect of rosuvastatin on low density lipoprotein cholesterol in patients with hypercholesterolaemia. *Am J Cardiol* 2001;88:504-08.
56. Davidson M, Ma P, Stein EA et al. Comparison of effects of low-density lipoprotein cholesterol and high density lipoprotein cholesterol with rosuvastatin versus atorvastatin with type IIa or IIb hyper-cholesterolaemia. *Am J Cardiol* 2002;89:268-75.
57. Paoletti R, Fahmy M, Mahla G et al. ZD4522 is superior to pravastatin and simvastatin in reducing LDL cholesterol, enabling more hyper-cholesterolaemic patients to achieve target LDL guidelines. *J Am Coll Cardiol* 2001;37(Suppl): 291A (abs174).
58. Farnier M. Ezetimibe in hypercholesterolaemia. *Int J Clin Prac* 2002;56:8.
59. Bays HE, Moore PB, Drehobl MA et al. Effectiveness and tolerability of ezetimibe in patients with primary hypercholesterolemia: pooled analysis of two phase II studies. *Clin Ther* 2001;23:1209-30.
60. Knopp RH, Gitter H, Truitt T et al. Ezetimibe reduces low density lipoprotein cholesterol: results of a phase III randomised, double-blind, placebo-controlled trial. *Atherosclerosis* 2001;2(Suppl 2):38 (abs).
61. Dujovne CA, Ettinger MP, McNeer JF et al. Ezetimibe, a selective cholestrol absorption inhibitor, improves plasma lipids in hypercholesterolemic patients. *Circulation* 2001;104(Suppl II):176 (abs).
62. The Veterans Affairs High-Density Lipoprotein Cholesterol Intervention Trial Study Group. Gemfibrozil for the secondary prevention of coronary heart disease in men with low levels of high-density lipoprotein cholesterol. *N Engl J Med* 1999;341:410-18.
63. Curb JD, Pressel SL, Cutler et al. Effect of diuretic-based antihypertensive treatment on cardiovascular disease risk in older diabetic patients with isolated systolic hypertension. Systolic Hypertension in the Elderly Program Cooperative Research Group. *JAMA* 1996;276:1886-92.
64. Tuomilehto J, Rastenyte D, Birkenhager WH et al. Effect of calcium-channel blockade in older subjects with diabetes and systolic hypertension. Systolic Hypertension in Europe Trial Investigators. *N Engl J Med* 1999;340:677-84.
65. Hansson L, Lindholm LH, Niskanen L et al. Effect of angiotensin-converting-enzyme inhibition compared with conventional therapy on cardiovascular morbidity and mortality in hypertension: the Captopril Prevention Project (CAPPP) randomised trial. *Lancet* 1999;3543:611-16.
66. Heart Outcomes Prevention Evaluation Study Investigators. Effects of ramipril on cardiovascular and microvascular outcomes in people with diabetes mellitus: results of the HOPE study and MICRO-HOPE sub-study. Heart Outcomes Prevention Evaluation Study Investigators. *Lancet* 2000;355:253-59.
67. Barnett AH. Pharmacology of antihypertensive drugs. In Barnett AH, Dodson PM (eds). *Hypertension and Diabetes* (3rd edn). London: Science Press Ltd 2000; 33-42.
68. Fusgen I, Schutz D. Use of indapamide SR in elderly patients in general practice. Results of a prospective study of 3,034 elderly multimorbid patients. *Eur J Ger* 2001;3(4):196-200.
69. Emeriau JP, Knauf H, Pujadas JO et al. A comparison of indapamide SR 1.5mg with both amlodipine 5mg and hydrochlorothiazide 25mg in elderly hypertensive patients: a randomised double-blind controlled study. *J Hypertension* 2001;19:343-50.
70. Leonetti G, Emeriau JP, Knauf H et al. Evaluation of long-term efficacy of indapamide SR 1.5mg in elderly hypertensive patients. *Am J Hypertension* 2001;14:4(Suppl 1):A102-A103.
71. Gosse P, Sheridan D, Zannad F et al. Regression of left ventricular hypertrophy in hypertensive patients treated with indapamide SR 1.5mg versus enalapril 20 mg: the LIVE study. *J Hypertension* 2000;18:1465-75.
72. Mallion J-M, Asmar R et al. Trough-to-peak ratio of indapamide 1.5 mg sustained-release coated tablets assessed by ambulatory blood pressure monitoring. *Archives des Maladies du Coeur et des Vaisseaux* 1996; Special issue: 2012.
73. Jaillon P, Asmar R, and the investigators of the 32-h ABPM Study. Thirty-two hour ambulatory blood pressure monitoring for the assessment of blood pressure evaluation in case of a missed dose of indapamide SR 1.5mg. European Society of Hypertension, Milan, 2001 (Abstract).

74. PROGRESS Collaborative Group. Randomised trial of a perindopril-based blood pressure lowering regimen among 6105 individuals with previous stroke or transient ischaemic attack. *Lancet* 2001;358:1033-41.
75. ALLHAT Collaborative Research Group. Major outcomes in high risk, hypertensive, patients randomised to angiotensin converting enzyme inhibitor or calcium channel blocker versus diuretic. *J Am Med Assoc* 2002;288:2981-97.
76. Brown JJ, Casals-Stenzel J, Cumming AMM et al. Angiotensin II, aldosterone and arterial pressure: a quantitative approach. *Hypertension* 1979;1:159-79.
77. Parving HH, Lehnert H, Brochner-Mortensen J et al; Irbesartan in patients with type 2 diabetes and microalbuminuria study group. The effect of irbesartan on the development of diabetic nephropathy in patients with type 2 diabetes. *N Engl J Med* 2001;345:870-78.
78. Lewis EJ, Hunsicker LG, Clarke WR et al; collaborative study group. Renoprotective effect of the angiotensin-receptor antagonist irbesartan in patients with nephropathy due to type 2 diabetes. *N Engl J Med* 2001;345:851-60.
79. Brenner BM, Cooper ME, de Zeeuw D et al; RENAAL study investigators. Effect of losartan on renal and cardiovascular outcomes in patients with type 2 diabetes and nephropathy. *N Engl J Med* 2001;345:861-69.
80. Dahlof B, Devereux RB, Kjeldsen SE et al. Cardiovascular morbidity and mortality in the Losartan Intervention For Endpoint reduction in hypertension study (LIFE): a randomised trial against atenolol. *Lancet* 2002;359:995-1003.
81. Pfeffer MA, Swedberg K, Granger CB et al. Effects of candesartan on mortality and morbidity in patients with chronic heart failure: the CHARM-Overall programme. *Lancet* 2003;363:759-66.
82. McMurray JJV, Ostergren J, Swedberg K et al. Effects of candesartan in patients with chronic heart failure and reduced left-ventricular systolic function taking aniotensin-converting-enzyme inhibitors: the CHARM-Added trial. *Lancet* 2003;362:767-71.
83. Granger CB, McMurray JJV, Yusuf S et al. Effects of candesartan in patients with chronic heart failure and reduced left-ventricular systolic function intolerant to angiotensin-converting-enzyme inhibitors: the CHARM-Alternative trial. *Lancet* 2003;362:772-76.
84. Yusuf S, Pfeffer MA, Swedberg K et al. Effects of candesartan in patients with chronic heart failure and preserved left-ventricular ejection fraction: the CHARM-Preserved Trial. *Lancet* 2003;362: 777-81.
85. White HD. Commentary. Candesartan and heart failure: the allure of CHARM. *Lancet* 2003; 362: 754-55.
86. The DCCT Research Group. The effects of intensive treatment of diabetes on the development and progression of long-term complications in insulin-dependent diabetes mellitus. *N Eng J Med* 1993; 329:977-86.
87. Bailey CJ. Antidiabetic drugs. *Br J Cardiol* 2000;7: 350-60.
88. Effect of intensive blood-glucose control with metformin on complications in overweight patients with type 2 diabetes (UKPDS 34). *Lancet* 1998;353: 854-65.
89. Lebovitz HE. Alpha-glucosidase inhibitors as agents in the treatment of diabetes. *Diabetes Rev* 1998;6: 132-45.
90. Davies MJ. Insulin secretagogues. In: Barnett AH (ed). *Current Medical Research and Opinion in Diabetes Mellitus*. Newbury, UK: Librapharm, 2002;18 Suppl 1:S22-30.
91. Horton E, Clinkingbeard C, Gatlin M et al. Nateglinide alone and in combination with metformin improves glycaemic control by reducing mealtime glucose levels in type 2 diabetes. *Diabetes Care* 2000;23:1660-65.
92. DECODE Study Group on behalf of the European Diabetes Epidemiology Study Group. Glucose tolerance and mortality: comparison of WHO and American Diabetes Association diagnostic criteria. *Lancet* 1999;354:617-21.
93. Hanefeld M, Dickinson S, Bouter KP et al. Rapid and short-acting mealtime insulin secretion with nateglinide controls both prandial and mean glycaemia. *Diabetes Care* 2000;23:2:202-07.
94. Barnett AH. Insulin-sensitising agents – thiazolidinediones (glitazones). *Curr Med Res Opin* 2002;18 (Suppl):31s-9.
95. Barman Balfour JA, Plosker GL. Rosiglitazone. *Drugs* 1999;57:921-30.
96. Matthews DR, Bakst A, Weston WM et al. Rosiglitazone decreases insulin resistance and improves beta-cell function in patients with type 2 diabetes. Abstr. 858. The 35th Annual Meeting of the European Association for the Study of Diabetes. *Diabetologia* 1999;42(Suppl 1):228.
97. Einhorn D, Rendell M, Rosenzweig J, et al. Pioglitazone hydrochloride in combination with metformin in the treatment of type 2 diabetes mellitus: a randomized, placebo-controlled study. The Pioglitazone 027 Study Group. *Clin Ther* 2000; 22(12):1395-409.
98. Kipnes MS, Krosnick A, Rendell MS. Pioglitazone hydrochloride in combination with sulfonylurea therapy improves glycemic control in patients with

type 2 diabetes mellitus: a randomized, placebo-controlled study. *Am J Med* 2001; 111(1):10-17.
99. Hanefeld M, Göke B. Combining pioglitazone with a sulphonlyurea or metformin in the management of type 2 diabetes. *Exp Clin Endocrinol Diabetes* 2000; 108 (Suppl 2): S256-S266.
100. Bakris GL, Dole JF, Porter LA et al. Rosiglitazone improves blood pressure in patients with type 2 diabetes mellitus. *Diabetes* 2000;49(Suppl 1): 388 (abs).
101. Pavo I, Jermendy G, Varkonyi TT et al. Effect of pioglitazone compared with metformin on glycemic control and indicators of insulin sensitivity in recently diagnosed patients with type 2 diabetes. J Clin Endocrinol Metab 2003;88(4):1637-45.
102. Raskin P, Dole JE, Rappaport EB. Rosiglitazone improves glycaemic control in poorly controlled insulin-treated type 2 diabetes (T2D). *Diabetes* 1999;48(Suppl 1):A94.
103. Barnett AH. A review of basal insulin. D*iabetic Med* 2003; 20: 873-85.
104. Klonoff DC. Inhaled insulin. *Diabetes Technol Ther* 1999;1:307-13.
105. Barnett AH. Drug Profile. Pulmonary insulin delivery in type 1 and type 2 diabetes. *Future Prescriber* 2001;2:18-21.
106. Skyler JS, Cefalu WT, Kourides IA et al. Efficacy of inhaled insulin in type 1 diabetes mellitus: a randomised proof-of-concept study. *Lancet* 2001;357:331-35.
107. Weiss SR, Berger S, Cheng S-L et al. Adjunctive therapy with inhaled insulin type 2 diabetic patients failing oral agents: a multicenter phase II trial. *Diabetes* 1999;48(Suppl 1):A12.
108. Allahabadia A, Kumar S. Diabetes and obesity: what is the relationship to cardiovascular disease? In: Barnett AH (ed). *Diabetes Annual*. London: Martin Dunitz, 2002;15-39.
109. New GMS Contract - Supporting Documentation.The NHS Confederation 2003 (www.nhsconfed.org)
110. Testing Times. A Review of Diabetes Services in England and Wales. London: Audit Commission; 2000.
111. National Service Framework (NSF) for Diabetes: Standards. London: Department of Health 2001.
112. O'Gara MG. Integrated care – strengthening hospital and community links in the management of people with diabetes. *Mod Diabetes Manage* 2000;1(3):2-5.

Index